T0210252

Management of Obesity, Part 2: Treatment Strategies

Editors

AMANDA VELAZQUEZ
LEE M. KAPLAN

GASTROENTEROLOGY CLINICS OF NORTH AMERICA

www.gastro.theclinics.com

Consulting Editor
ALAN L. BUCHMAN

December 2023 • Volume 52 • Number 4

ELSEVIER

1600 John F. Kennedy Boulevard • Suite 1800 • Philadelphia, Pennsylvania, 19103-2899
http://www.theclinics.com

GASTROENTEROLOGY CLINICS OF NORTH AMERICA Volume 52, Number 4
December 2023 ISSN 0889-8553, ISBN-13: 978-0-323-94013-9

Editor: Kerry Holland
Developmental Editor: Isha Singh

Gastroenterology Clinics of North America (ISSN 0889-8553) is published quarterly by Elsevier Inc., 360 Park Avenue South, New York, NY 10010-1710. Months of issue are March, June, September, and December. Business and Editorial Offices: 1600 John F. Kennedy Blvd., Suite 1800, Philadelphia, PA 19103-2899. Customer Service Office: 6277 Sea Harbor Drive, Orlando, FL 32887-4800. Periodicals postage paid at New York, NY and additional mailing offices. Subscription prices are $379.00 per year (US individuals), $100.00 per year (US students), $849.00 per year (US institutions), $407.00 per year (Canadian individuals), $100.00 per year (Canadian students), $1041.00 per year (Canadian institutions), $482.00 per year (international individuals), $220.00 per year (international students), and $1041.00 per year (international institutions). Foreign air speed delivery is included in all *Clinics* subscription prices. All prices are subject to change without notice. **POSTMASTER**: Send address changes to *Gastroenterology Clinics of North America*, Elsevier Health Sciences Division, Subscription Customer Service, 3251 Riverport Lane, Maryland Heights, MO 63043. **Telephone: 1-800-654-2452 (U.S. and Canada); 314-447-8871 (outside U.S. and Canada). Fax: 314-447-8029. E-mail: journalscustomerservice-usa@elsevier.com (for print support); journalsonlinesupport-usa@elsevier.com (for online support).**

Reprints. For copies of 100 or more, of articles in this publication, please contact the Commercial Reprints Department, Elsevier Inc., 360 Part Avenue South, New York, New York 10010-1710. Tel. 212-633-3874, Fax: 212-633-3820, E-mail: reprints@elsevier.com.

Gastroenterology Clinics of North America is also published in Italian by Il Pensiero Scientifico Editore, Rome, Italy; and in Portuguese by Interlivros Edicoes Ltda., Rua Commandante Coelho 1085, 21250 Cordovil, Rio de Janeiro, Brazil.

Gastroenterology Clinics of North America is covered in *MEDLINE/PubMed (Index Medicus), Excerpta Medica, Current Contents/Clinical Medicine, Science Citation Index, ISI/BIOMED*, and *BIOSIS*.

Contributors

CONSULTING EDITOR

ALAN L. BUCHMAN, MD, MSPH, FACP, FACN, FACG, AGAF
Professor of Clinical Surgery, Medical Director, Intestinal Rehabilitation and Transplant Center, The University of Illinois at Chicago, UI Health, Chicago, Illinois, USA

EDITORS

AMANDA VELAZQUEZ, MD, DABOM
Associate Professor of Surgery and Medicine, Director of Obesity Medicine, Department of General Surgery, Center for Weight Management and Metabolic Health, Cedars-Sinai Medical Center, Los Angeles, California, USA

LEE M. KAPLAN, MD, PhD
Director, Boston Course in Obesity Medicine, The Obesity and Metabolism Institute, Massachusetts General Hospital, Boston, Massachusetts, USA

AUTHORS

BARHAM K. ABU DAYYEH, MD, MPH
Department of Gastroenterology and Hepatology, Mayo Clinic, Rochester, Minnesota, USA

KHALED ALABDULJABBAR, MD
Diabetes Complications Research Centre, Conway Institute, University College Dublin, Dublin, Ireland; Department of Family Medicine and Polyclinics, King Faisal Specialist Hospital and Research Centre, Riyadh, Saudi Arabia

LOUIS J. ARONNE, MD, FACP, DABOM
Sanford I. Weill Professor of Metabolic Research, Director, Comprehensive Weight Control Center at Weill Cornell Medicine, Division of Endocrinology, Diabetes and Metabolism, NewYork-Presbyterian Hospital, Weill Cornell Medical College, Comprehensive Weight Control Center, New York, New York, USA

SARAH R. BARENBAUM, MD, DABOM
Assistant Professor of Clinical Medicine, Division of Endocrinology, Diabetes and Metabolism, NewYork-Presbyterian Hospital, Weill Cornell Medical College, Comprehensive Weight Control Center, New York, New York, USA

EFSTATHIOS BONANOS, MD
Altnagelvin Hospital, Londonderry, United Kingdom

VITOR BRUNALDI, MD, PhD
Department of Gastroenterology and Hepatology, Mayo Clinic, Rochester, Minnesota, USA

ALISON R. FORTE, BA
Division of Pediatric Endocrinology and Diabetes, Department of Pediatrics, Icahn School of Medicine at Mount Sinai, New York, New York, USA

KHUSHBOO GALA, MBBS
Department of Gastroenterology and Hepatology, Mayo Clinic, Rochester, Minnesota, USA

JOAN C. HAN, MD
Professor of Pediatrics, Division of Pediatric Endocrinology and Diabetes, Department of Pediatrics, Icahn School of Medicine at Mount Sinai, New York, New York, USA; Departments of Pediatrics and Physiology, The University of Tennessee Health Sciences Center, Memphis, Tennessee, USA

ANDREA M. HAQQ, MD
Department of Pediatrics, Faculty of Medicine and Dentistry, Department of Agricultural, Food and Nutritional Science, University of Alberta, Edmonton, Alberta, Canada

KELVIN HIGA, MD, FACS, FASMBS, FIFSO
Clinical Professor, University of California San Francisco, Co-Director, ALSA Minimally Invasive-Bariatric Surgery Fellowship Program, and Medical Director, Minimally Invasive and Bariatric Surgery Program, Fresno Heart & Surgical Hospital, Fresno, California, USA

SCOTT KAHAN, MD, MPH
George Washington University School of Medicine, National Center for Weight and Wellness, Washington, DC, USA

REKHA B. KUMAR, MD, MS, DABOM
Associate Professor of Clinical Medicine, Iris Cantor Women's Health Center, Endocrinology and Internal Medicine, New York, New York, USA

THEODORE K. KYLE, RPH, MBA
Principal and Founder, ConscienHealth, Pittsburgh, Pennsylvania, USA

CAREL W. LE ROUX, PhD
Diabetes Complications Research Centre, Conway Institute, University College Dublin, Dublin, Ireland

ALEXANDER D. MIRAS, PhD
School of Medicine, Ulster University, Londonderry, United Kingdom

JOE NADGLOWSKI, BS
President and CEO, Obesity Action Coalition, Tampa, Florida, USA

MARCUS C. RASMUSSEN, BA
Division of Pediatric Endocrinology and Diabetes, Department of Pediatrics, Icahn School of Medicine at Mount Sinai, New York, New York, USA

JOHN H. RODRIGUEZ, MD
Department of General Surgery, Cleveland Clinic Abu Dhabi, Al Maryah Island, United Arab Emirates

DONNA H. RYAN, MD
Professor Emerita, Pennington Biomedical Research Center, Baton Rouge, Louisiana, USA

SARAH H. SCHMITZ, MD
Instructor in Medicine, Division of Endocrinology, Diabetes and Metabolism, NewYork-Presbyterian Hospital, Weill Cornell Medical College, Comprehensive Weight Control Center, New York, New York, USA

STEPHANIE B. SCHRAGE, BA
Division of Pediatric Endocrinology and Diabetes, Department of Pediatrics, Icahn School of Medicine at Mount Sinai, New York, New York, USA

JOSHUA S. WINDER, MD
Division of Minimally Invasive and Bariatric Surgery, Penn State Milton S. Hershey Medical Center, Hershey, Pennsylvania, USA

SARAH K. ZAFAR, BA
Division of Pediatric Endocrinology and Diabetes, Department of Pediatrics, Icahn School of Medicine at Mount Sinai, New York, New York, USA

Contents

GASTROENTEROLOGY CLINICS OF NORTH AMERICA

FORTHCOMING ISSUES

March 2024
Pathology of Dysplasia in the Gastrointestinal Tract
Robert Odze, *Editor*

June 2024
Advances in Intestinal Transplantation, Part I
Alan L. Buchman, *Editor*

September 2024
Advances in Intestinal Transplantation, Part II
Alan L. Buchman, *Editor*

RECENT ISSUES

September 2023
Pediatric Inflammatory Bowel Disease
Marla Dubinsky, *Editor*

June 2023
Management of Obesity, Part I: Overview and Basic Mechanisms
Lee M. Kaplan, *Editor*

March 2023
COVID-19 and Gastroenterology
Mitchell S. Cappell, *Editor*

SERIES OF RELATED INTEREST

Clinics in Liver Disease
(https://www.liver.theclinics.com)
Gastrointestinal Endoscopy Clinics of North America
(https://www.giendo.theclinics.com)

Preface

Comprehensive Treatment Approaches To Obesity

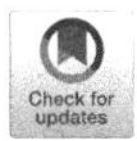

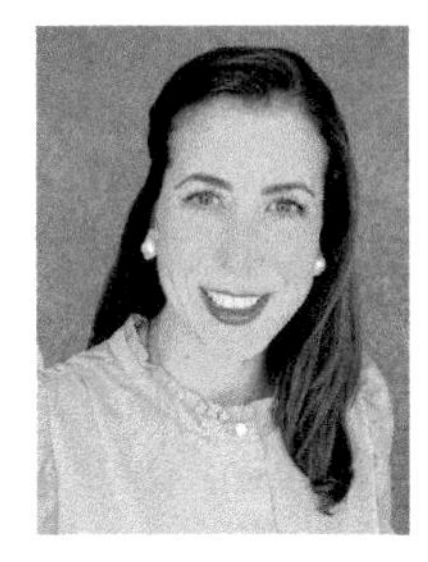

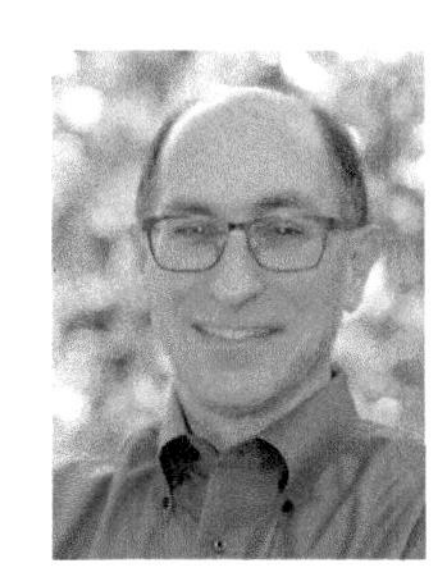

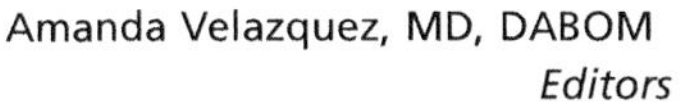
Amanda Velazquez, MD, DABOM Lee M. Kaplan, MD, PhD
Editors

This issue of *Gastroenterology Clinics of North America* provides a comprehensive overview of the spectrum of existing approaches for obesity treatment. Obesity is a complex, chronic disease that is critical to address with a multidisciplinary, bias-free approach. Ideally treatments should begin upstream so as to prevent the numerous weight-related medical conditions, including cardiovascular disease, type 2 diabetes, cancer, and more. While lifestyle modifications remain the foundation for treating obesity, these methods alone have proven insufficient for the majority of patients to improve health through sustained, long-term weight loss. As a result, additional treatment modalities are often indicated, such as pharmacotherapy, advanced endoscopic procedures, and bariatric surgery.

The expert authors in this issue aim to elucidate the research behind the various treatment approaches and explore the foundations of obesity treatment, emphasizing the pivotal role of lifestyle modifications. This includes healthy eating, physical activity, and behavioral interventions. Since obesity is a heterogenous disease, the response to any treatment, including lifestyle modification, will vary. Here are also numerous subtypes of obesity, including those of genetic cause, like monogenic and syndromic obesity. Identifying these rare conditions and considering targeted medication treatment are critical. Some individuals are even affected by medication-induced weight gain. There must be a greater awareness by health care professionals to determine the risk of weight gain considered against the benefits of the medication at hand. Fortunately, there are often medication alternatives that can be considered to promote weight loss, many of which are used on- or off-label for the treatment of obesity.

Authors review the evolving landscape of pharmacologic treatments of obesity, including the mechanisms of action and potential benefits, while also discussing limitations and side effects. Antiobesity medications are used for both nonsurgical and

Gastroenterol Clin N Am 52 (2023) xi–xii
https://doi.org/10.1016/j.gtc.2023.09.008
0889-8553/23/© 2023 Published by Elsevier Inc.

surgical patients, and authors address their utility for weight regain after bariatric surgery. The heart of this issue delves into a balanced overview of the surgical obesity treatments, beginning with the fundamentals of bariatric surgery and its mechanism of action on body weight regulation, followed by analysis of surgical complications and their management. The emerging field of endoscopic treatment of obesity is discussed along with ways to identify which patients may be the best candidates. Finally, authors examine the need for shared decision making and bias-free language when discussing obesity and obesity treatments with patients. Because obesity ultimately is an individualized journey, precision medicine is required to find the most suitable and sustainable approach to each patient's unique weight management needs.

DISCLOSURES

Board Member/Advisory Panel: Weight Watchers, Intellihealth; Consultant: Novo Nordisk; Research Support: NIH Grant, National Heart, Lung, and Blood Institute (NCT0517662), UCLA Clinical and Translational Science Institute (CSTI) Grant.

Amanda Velazquez, MD, DABOM
Department of General Surgery
Center for Weight Management and Metabolic Health
Cedars-Sinai Medical Center
8635 West 3rd Street, #795W
Los Angeles, CA 90048, USA

Lee M. Kaplan, MD, PhD
The Obesity and Metabolism Institute
Massachusetts General Hospital
55 Fruit Street
Boston, MA 02114, USA

E-mail addresses:
Amanda.Velazquez@cshs.org (A. Velazquez)
lmkaplan@partners.org (L.M. Kaplan)

Lifestyle-Based Obesity Care

Donna H. Ryan, MD

KEYWORDS

- Lifestyle intervention • Dietary intervention • Physical activity intervention
- Chronic weight management • Weight loss • Weight loss maintenance
- Intensive behavioral therapy for obesity

KEY POINTS

- Lifestyle intervention—the implementation of changes in behavior around diet and physical activity—is foundational to any weight loss effort, whether using medications, devices, or surgical approaches.
- The evidence of health benefits from lifestyle intervention was derived from interventions delivered in face-to-face (group or individual) sessions, with at least 14 sessions over 6 months and continued follow-up provided to 1 year and produced average weight loss of 8 kg at 1 year. This is the "gold-standard" intervention.
- It is difficult to implement the evidence-based lifestyle interventions recommended by guidelines, and real-world studies using embedded health coaches show more modest weight loss.
- Even with intensive lifestyle intervention delivered to a gold standard, not all patients can achieve weight loss, and weight regain is common.

INTRODUCTION AND BACKGROUND

Personal attempts to lose weight by adults are a common phenomenon around the globe. In a systematic review and meta-analysis of 72 studies that included more than 1 million adults, 42% of adults from general populations were trying to lose weight by exercise and dieting and 22% were trying to maintain weight.[1] Across these studies, higher prevalence of weight loss attempts was found in women and in individuals with overweight and obesity as compared with normal weight. The methods used to lose weight in these studies included a variety of diets and increasing physical activity. In the face of the widespread efforts to lose weight, there is the increasing prevalence of obesity, worldwide.[2] In the United States the latest nationally representative survey of adults showed that the prevalence of body mass index (BMI) 30 kg/m^2 was 42.4%.[3] Given the public health implications of this degree of disease burden in the population, a public health response with lifestyle intervention is indicated.

Pennington Biomedical Research Center, 6400 Perkins Road, Baton Rouge, LA 70808, USA
E-mail address: ryandh@pbrc.edu

Gastroenterol Clin N Am 52 (2023) 645–660
https://doi.org/10.1016/j.gtc.2023.08.001

US Preventive Services Task Force's latest recommendation from 2018 states, "the USPSTF recommends that clinicians offer or refer adults with a body mass index of 30 or higher to intensive, multicomponent behavioral interventions. (B recommendation)".[4] It should be noted that the interventions that formed the basis for the evidence that supports the USPSTF recommendation in most cases did not include the physician or health care provider in the intervention, hence the "offer or refer." Achieving weight loss in the medical office setting has been challenging, as described later (**Box 1**).

The American Heart Association/American College of Cardiology/The Obesity Society (AHA/ACC/TOS) Guideline's systematic evidence review[5] of lifestyle intervention demonstrated that when lessons to change behaviors around diet and physical activity were delivered in face-to-face (group or individual) sessions, with at least 14 sessions over 6 months and continued follow-up is provided to 1 year, then average weight loss of 8 kg weight loss at 1 year is the result. Although this may seem modest weight loss, it translates into clinically significant improvements in blood pressure, triglycerides, high-density lipoprotein cholesterol, measures of glycemic control, and reduction in risk for progression to type 2 diabetes.[5] In these recommendations, intensive behavioral therapy is comprehensive, that is, addressing behaviors around both food intake and physical activity.

A fundamental tenet of all guidance and recommendations for obesity management is that lifestyle intervention—changing behaviors around diet and physical activity—is foundational; that is, all other approaches with medications, devices, and surgery rest on lifestyle changes; this is true for the AHA/ACC/TOS Guidelines,[5] the American Association of Clinical Endocrinology Guidelines,[6] the Endocrine Guidelines about pharmacotherapy,[7] and the guidelines for bariatric surgery.[8] With lifestyle as the foundation for successful weight loss with adjunctive therapies, it is essential that health care professionals understand what contributes to success in lifestyle intervention.

DISCUSSION

Creating an Energy Deficit

The mechanism behind weight loss is straightforward: to lose one pound, one must create an energy deficit of 3500 kcal (to lose 1 kg, one must create an energy deficit of 7700 kcal [32.2 mJ]).[9] This assumes that the individual has 30 kg or more body fat, as is the case in obesity; if leaner, the energy requirements would be somewhat less because of the composition of body fat loss.[9] The energy deficit occurs by increasing energy expenditure through physical activity or by reducing energy intake through dieting.

Predicting Weight Loss

Energy requirements to maintain weight can be calculated based on age, sex, weight, height, and physical activity level. Several of the most used formulae to calculate this are the Harris Benedict equation, the Mifflin St Jeor equation, or the FAO/WHO/UNU equation.[10–12] Most often individuals who are using the measurement of energy requirements to calculate weight loss on an energy deficit diet will use an online Body

Box 1

The USPSTF recommends that clinicians offer or refer adults with a body mass index of 30 kg/m^2 or higher to intensive, multicomponent behavioral interventions (B recommendation).[4]

Weight Planner, such as that sponsored by the National Institutes of Health (NIH) https://www.niddk.nih.gov/bwp that incorporates these formulae.

Setting the Weight Loss Goal and Tracking Success

In all lifestyle interventions, the coach and patient set specific, attainable goals and track progress; this is true for all the behaviors one is hoping to modify, and use of food diaries and exercise trackers is essential, as is tracking weight. There are many body weight planners available for use on the Internet. One of the best is the NIH Body Weight Planner mentioned earlier and found at https://www.niddk.nih.gov/bwp. **Fig. 1** shows how the Body Weight Planner can be used to create an expected weight loss over a defined period by modifying energy intake and energy expenditure.

Defining the Goal and Expectations

For lifestyle intervention, an initial goal is usually 10% to be achieved over 6 months and maintained for 1 year.[5] It is unusual for patients to be able to achieve and sustain greater amounts of weight loss without adding ancillary therapy with drugs, devices, or surgery.[5]

Learning from "Gold-Standard" Interventions

The endorsement of lifestyle intervention by the USPSTF and multiple guidelines rests primarily on several large, long-term studies of lifestyle intervention for weight loss, primarily Diabetes Prevention Program,[13–15] and Look AHEAD.[16–19] These large randomized clinical trials were conducted in multiple academic health centers and

Body Weight Planner | Balancing Your Food and Activity
Step 2 of 4 - Enter your goal weight
Step 3 of 4 - Enter your physical activity change (optional)
Step 4 of 4 - Results
Weight Goal
Goal Weight 167 lbs
I want to reach my goal in 187 days
OR select a date
I want to reach my goal by 2/15/2023
Physical Activity Change
To reach my goal, I will change my physical activity by 15 %
Results
Weight
Sex
Age
Height
Physical Activity Level
In order to maintain your current weight, you should eat: 2,349 Calories/day
To reach your goal of 169 lbs in 180 days, you should eat: 2,013 Calories/day
To maintain your goal of 169 lbs. you should eat: 2,322 Calories/day
Estimate Percent Change in Physical Activity Level
I will make the following changes to my physical activity:
Add
Medium Walking
30
5
week
This represents a change of 15% to your starting activity level

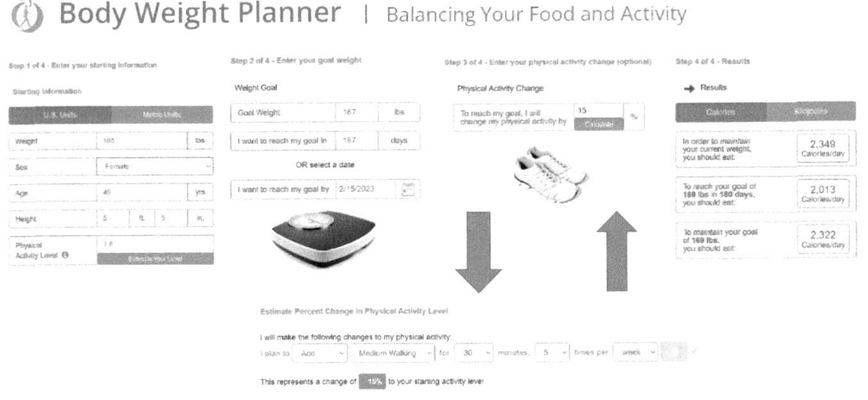

Fig. 1. Using a Body Weight Planner to calculate the trajectory of weight loss. Here we use the NIH Body Weight Planner for a hypothetical patient who is a woman, 49 years old, weighs 185 pounds, and has light activity at work and for recreation. This is entered into fields for Step 1. For Step 2, the goal weight and time point are determined. Here we select 10% weight loss (18 pounds lost to 167 pounds goal) by approximately 6 months (187 days). In Step 3, we first calculate the increase in physical activity by choosing an activity and indicating the duration and how often. We choose medium walking for 30 minutes 5 times a week. This tells us that the physical activity energy expenditure will increase by 15%. Finally, in Step 4 we see the calorie goal to achieve weight loss (2013 kcal daily in this case) and to maintain the lost weight at 169 pounds (2322 kcal/d). Example using Body Weight Planner courtesy of National Institute of Fiabetes and Digestive and Kidney Diseases, National Institutes of Health. https://www.niddk.nih.gob/bwp.

were not incorporated into routine practice. Delivering weight loss intervention in medical practices is difficult and produces on average only 1 to 3 kg weight loss.[19] Thus, 2 more recent studies, PROPEL[20,21] and REPOWER,[22,23] address this need for primary care approaches to obesity management and have been analyzed together.[24] **Table 1** describes these interventions.

As shown in **Table 1**, DPP[13–15] and Look AHEAD[16–19] were designed to test efficacy of lifestyle intervention. Indeed, the moderate weight loss in DPP had a major effect on prevention of diabetes progression in individuals with type 2 diabetes. There was a 58% reduction in progression to type 2 diabetes in the Intensive Lifestyle Intervention group compared with the support condition.[15] Although Look AHEAD did not demonstrate a reduction in cardiovascular events at 9.5 years of follow-up,[17] the Intensive Lifestyle Intervention did demonstrate many positive benefits on cardiovascular risk factors, use of medications, quality of life, and even cost benefits in terms of inpatient costs.[18,19]

Also shown in **Table 1** are PROPEL[20,21] and REPOWER.[22,23] These are pragmatic clinical trials, with interventions delivered in real-world settings, and the weight loss efficacy is less than that seen DPP and Look AHEAD. Thus, their more modest weight losses are more reflective of what can be achieved in primary care settings. The 2 studies differ in important ways.[24] Although both reflect real-world clinical practice settings, REPOWER was conducted primarily in rural settings in the mid-west US and PROPEL in lower income, primarily Black participants in Louisiana. Even more important, only one of the treatment assignments (PROPEL'S in-clinic individual visits) was like the fee-for-service model that is endorsed by Center for Medicare and Medicaid Services for reimbursement.[25] This Intensive Behavioral Therapy for Obesity (IBTO) can only be delivered by primary care health care providers to be eligible for reimbursement, not specialists such as gastroenterologists. Importantly, this intervention produced the least weight loss of all studied—2.6 kg at 2 years, and only 36% achieved 5% or more weight loss. Indeed, a narrative review of practice-based weight loss intervention supports that primary care providers are not currently delivering effective weight management approaches in clinical practice.[26] When primary care providers delivered brief behavioral counseling at monthly to quarterly visits, the average weight losses were 0.1 to 2.3 kg. The use of nurse practitioners and physician assistants to deliver the intervention seemed to improve outcomes, and the most promising approach for future development was deemed remotely delivered counseling with contacts > monthly (**Box 2**).

The "gold-standard" intensive lifestyle interventions have shown successful weight loss and associated health benefit in randomized clinical trials delivered in academic settings. It remains to be demonstrated that the health care setting of the medical office as currently configured can offer similar results with a fee-for-service reimbursement model.

Not Everyone Succeeds with Lifestyle Intervention

Even with the "gold-standard" intervention, not all participants achieved even modest weight loss. In Look AHEAD, 32% of participants did not achieve even 5% weight loss at 1 year.[18] Weight regain is also an issue, even with the "gold-standard" intervention. In Look AHEAD, there was weight regain beginning at year 1 in the intervention group. By 10 years there was less than a 3% weight difference in the intervention and control conditions.[19] These aspects of lifestyle intervention are serious limitations. Patients should be offered augmented therapy with medications, devices, or surgery to aid in long-term successful weight loss.

Table 1
Food intake, physical activity, and behavioral approaches in influential lifestyle intervention trials

	DPP[13–15]	Look AHEAD[16–19]	PROPEL[20,21]	REPOWER[22,23]
Baseline description of Lifestyle Intervention Participants	1079 participants with impaired glucose tolerance; mean age 50.6 y; mean BMI 33.6 kg/m^2	2570 participants with type 2 diabetes; mean age 58.6 y; mean BMI 26.3 kg/m^2 (women) and 35.3 kg/m^2 (men)	18 cluster randomized rural clinics serving low-income families; 803 participants; mean age 49.4 y; mean BMI 37.2 kg/m^2; 67.2% black; 25.8% diabetes; 66.5% < $40,000 annual income	36 cluster randomized clinics in rural settings tested 3 interventions—Medicare Intensive Behavior Therapy for Obesity (IBTO) fee-for-service model compared with in-clinic group visits and telephone-based group visits; with 1407 participants; mean age 54.7 y; mean BMI 36.7; 77% women; 0.5% black
Individual Goal	7% weight loss	10% weight loss	10% weight loss	—
Weight loss achieved in intervention group	Year 1 weight loss 7.2% Year 2 weight loss 5.8% Year 3 weight loss 4.5%	Year 1 weight loss 8.6% Year 4 weight loss 6.15%	Year 2 weight loss 4.99%	Mean weight loss at 24 mo was 2.6 kg in the in-clinic individual intervention (IBTO), 4.4 kg in the in-clinic group intervention, and 3.9 kg in the telephone group intervention
Diet quality	Reduce total dietary fat to <25% of calories; if weight loss was not achieved by lowering fat, calorie goals were introduced	≤30% total calories from fat (with ≤10% total calories from saturated fat) and ≥15% total calories from protein; liquid meal replacements (provided free of charge) and frozen food entrees and structured meal plans (conventional foods) for those who declined the meal replacements	Initial focus on portion-controlled foods with prepackaged foods and meal replacement shakes provided for first month. In collaboration with coaches, patients instructed in food purchase and preparation	Participants received a calorie goal (1200–1500 kcal/d if weight was <114 kg; 1500–1800 kcal/d if weight was ≥114 kg) and were instructed to consume a balanced diet with 5 or more fruit and vegetable servings per day. Portion control and optional use of protein shakes and frozen entrees were encouraged, but no food or scales were provided.

(*continued on next page*)

Table 1
(continued)

	DPP[13–15]	Look AHEAD[16–19]	PROPEL[20,21]	REPOWER[22,23]
Physical activity	Engage in and maintain moderate intensity activity, such as brisk walking, for at least 150 min/wk	Home-based exercise with gradual progression to goal of 175 min of moderate intensity physical activity per week	Increase physical activity gradually to 175 min/wk	Increase physical activity up to 225 min/wk, set weekly diet and physical activity goals, and self-monitor daily with a physical activity monitor and commercial app or written log
Curriculum	16 lessons in 6 mo, covering diet, exercise, and behavior modification; taught individually, face-to-face; then monthly individual and group sessions; toolbox approach	Based on DPP; 24 sessions in 6 mo; taught in 3 group and 1 individual sessions per month; after 6 mo, 2 group and 1 individual sessions for 1 y; toolbox approach from DPP	Delivered by clinic-based coaches; Based on DPP and Look AHEAD; weekly sessions (16 conducted in person and 6 conducted by telephone) in the first 6 mo, followed by sessions (alternating in-person visits and telephone calls) held at least monthly for the remaining 18 mo	IBTO: 15-min in-clinic individual visits at a frequency similar to that reimbursed by Medicare (weekly for 1 mo, biweekly for 5 mo, and monthly thereafter). For the in-clinic group intervention, practice-employed clinicians delivered group visits weekly for 3 mo, biweekly for 3 mo, and monthly thereafter. All based on Look AHEAD intervention.

Behavioral techniques	Self-monitoring of weight, dietary intake, and physical activity; Regular meal pattern; Eating slowly; Stimulus control; Label reading; Contingency planning	Self-monitoring of weight, dietary intake, and physical activity; Regular meal pattern; Eating slowly; Stimulus control; Label reading; contingency planning. Orlistat optional after 6 mo	Self-monitoring of weight, dietary intake, and physical activity; Regular meal pattern; Eating slowly; Stimulus control; Label reading; contingency planning. Patients given scale that registered electronically to weight loss planner that graphically displayed weight loss trajectory. Educational materials were health literacy and culturally appropriate	Self-monitoring of weight, dietary intake, and physical activity; Regular meal pattern; Eating slowly; Stimulus control; Label reading; contingency planning. Patients encouraged to use Lose it! app
Health benefits associated with the intervention	Diabetes prevention: 58% reduction in progression from impaired glucose tolerance to type 2 diabetes after about 3 y as compared with control condition	After 9.5 y, no difference in cardiovascular event rate compared with control condition; improved biomarkers of glucose and lipid control, less sleep apnea, lower liver fat, less depression, improved insulin sensitivity, less urinary incontinence, less kidney disease, reduced need of diabetes medications, maintenance of physical mobility, improved quality of life and lower health care costs[19]	Changes in cardiometabolic risk factors were minimal and consistent with the modest degree of weight loss at 1 and 2 y. There were some improvements in quality-of-life measures with the modest weight loss in the intervention group as compared with usual care	No cardiometabolic risk factors reported; proportion achieving 5% weight loss (44.1%, 41.4%, 36%) was not significant among the 3 conditions. Similarly for 10% weight loss (22.6%, 22.3%, 17.1%) difference was not significant

Box 2

Center for Medicare and Medicaid Services will reimburse for Intensive Behavioral Therapy for Obesity (IBTO) when delivered by primary care providers (not specialists).[25] However, provision of weight loss counseling in a fee-for-service model with brief health care provider counseling has not been shown to produce effective weight loss.[22,26]

Behavioral Components of the Lifestyle Intervention

The cornerstone of treatment is self-monitoring, which means that patients must be trained to record food and calorie intake, physical activity, and various health parameters related to obesity (ie, body weight, waist circumference, blood pressure, and so on); this may be done electronically or with paper and pencil. The interventionist reviews records and with the patient targets areas for change and provides reinforcement of positive behaviors. Problem-solving is a skill set taught to identify challenges and solutions. Stimulus control refers to altering the patient's environment to remove food cues from the environment that sabotage dietary adherence and to promote activity-related and eating-related cues that are healthier. Eating slowly and extending the time of chewing promotes mindfulness and allows time for satiety signals to act and promotes reduction in food intake. Patients are taught label reading to promote intake of healthier food choices and to track caloric intake. Contingency planning allows individuals to plan ahead to promote adherence to lifestyle changes. Mindfulness training promotes greater awareness of body cues, satiety, hunger, and external cues related to the eating environment. Further information on these behavioral techniques used in the DPP and Look AHEAD are available in those intervention descriptions.[14,16]

Role of Health Care Professional in Offering or Referring for Lifestyle Intervention

As part of Look AHEAD, all interventionists were trained in motivational interviewing. This technique emerged from addiction counseling, engages the patient in resolving ambivalence, and has aids in weight loss.[27] Although physicians may delegate the role of interventionist to a nurse practitioner of physician's assistant, the patient must be engaged in decision-making around behavior change for success.

Referral for Intensive Lifestyle Intervention—Commercial Options and Community Programs

The estimated value of the US weight loss industry is $75 billion in 2022.[28] Given the difficulty of achieving successful weight loss in the medical office, referral is a reasonable option. A recent review[29] provides the relevant evidence supporting guidelines-bases commercial programs.

Community Programs

For patients with prediabetes community National DPP programs are available. Based on the evidence from the DPP[15] in prevention conversion from impaired glucose tolerance to type 2 diabetes, the Centers for Disease Control established the National DPP in 2010.[30] Patients must be living with overweight or obesity and meet risk criteria for type 2 diabetes, criteria that can be established online.[30] There are more than 1500 programs available, and their location can be identified online by relationship to a zipcode.[31] The program is covered by Medicare and some employer-based insurers.[32]

Box 3

Referral to community or commercial lifestyle programs is acceptable. Intervention can be delivered face-to-face or electronically and should continue for 1 year or more.

Commercial Programs

In the recent review,[29] commercial weight management programs were identified that delivered programs according to guideline recommendations.[5] This review found that "among the guideline-concordant programs, National Diabetes Prevention Program, WW, Jenny Craig, Medifast and OPTIFAST have demonstrated 12-month weight-loss efficacy and safety."[29] The review used evidence from randomized controlled trials to support this statement. Of these programs, National DPP is discussed earlier. WW (formerly known as Weight Watchers) offers lifestyle intervention in person or online through Web portal or app. Jenny Craig provides telephone counseling and

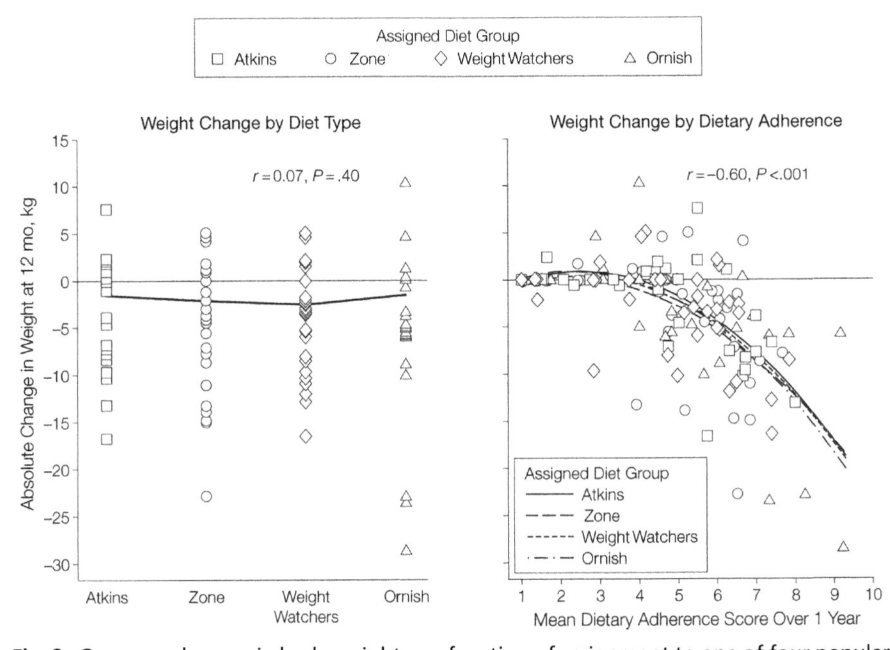

Fig. 2. One-year changes in body weight as a function of assignment to one of four popular diets and dietary adherence level for all study participants. Each study participant's weight change from baseline is shown in the panel at left. The line represents average weight loss, which is similar across the 4 diets. There is great variability in weight loss response for each of the 4 popular diets. There was no significant association between diet type and weight loss ($r = 0.07$; $P = .40$). In the panel at right, the mean dietary adherence over a year is plotted against weight loss. There is strong curvilinear association between self-reported dietary adherence and weight loss ($r = 0.60$; $P < .001$) that was almost identical for each diet. The curve in the weight change by diet type plot indicates the Lowes regression function, a locally weighted, least-squares method using 3 iterations to fit the data. The curves in the weight change by dietary adherence plot indicate the quadratic regression functions for each diet group. (*From* Dansinger ML, Gleason JA, Griffith JL, Selker HP, SchaeferEJ, Comparison of the Atkins, Ornish, Weight Watchers, and Zone diets for weight loss and heart disease risk reduction: a randomized trial. JAMA.2005 jan 5;293(1):43 to 53; with permission.)

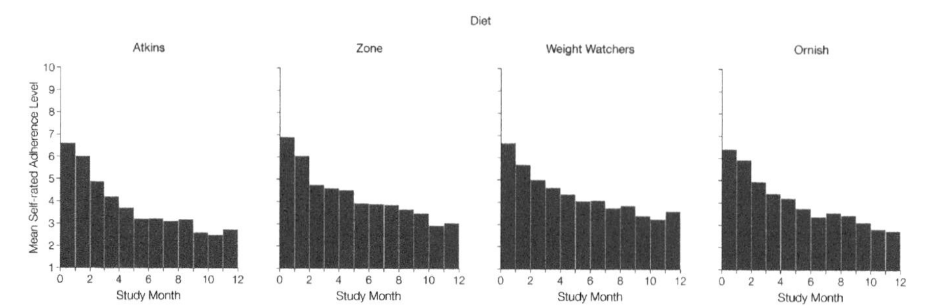

Fig. 3. Adherence to four popular diets wanes over 1 year. Each month during the study, participants self-rated adherence to the diet from 1 (none) to 10 (perfect). Across all 4 diets there was a reduction in adherence that increased over time. Baseline values were carried forward in cases of missing data. Range of standard deviation for all 4 diet groups was from 1.9 to 3.5. (*From* Dansinger ML, Gleason JA, Griffith JL, Selker HP, SchaeferEJ, Comparison of the Atkins, Ornish, Weight Watchers, and Zone diets for weight loss and heart disease risk reduction: a randomized trial. JAMA.2005 jan 5;293(1):43 to 53; with permission.)

provision of food. Medifast and Optifast are meal replacement programs providing low-calorie (800–1200 kcal/d) or very-low-calorie (<800 kcal/day) diets. Although HMR and Nutrisystem provide meal replacement approaches, they did not report 12-month data. This review noted that Web-based or virtual programs are emerging, and Noom and Omada Health have ongoing randomized clinical trials that may support their efficacy.[29]

Dietary Intervention

In a 2021 survey, 39% of Americans reported having followed a specific diet or eating pattern within the past year, most for weight loss or weight maintenance.[33] The top strategies were calorie counting (10%), clean eating (9%)—this refers to eating unprocessed foods—intermittent fasting (8%), ketogenic or high-fat diet (5%), and low-carb diet (6%).[33] Despite the continued popularity of dieting to lose weight, with ever-changing fads, guidelines teach us that there are multiple dietary pathways to successful weight loss.[5] In fact of the 18 dietary approaches subjected to systematic evidence review for the Obesity Guidelines,[5] no one dietary approach was superior in terms of weight loss (**Box 3**).

A 2002 study of 4 popular diets is informative.[34] In that study, 160 adults with overweight or obesity and cardiovascular risk factor abnormalities were randomly assigned to 1 of 4 diets: Atkins (a carbohydrate restriction diet), Zone (macronutrient balance), Weight Watchers (calorie restriction), or Ornish (fat restriction diet). There were 40 individuals in each group.

In **Fig. 2**, individual weight loss in kilogram is depicted for every participant at 1 year. The average weight loss is shown in the line. There is no difference in average weight loss by diet (p for trend 0.40). The average kilogram (standard deviation) lost at 1 year is Atkins 2.1 (4.8), Zone −3.2 (6.0), Weight Watchers −3.0 (4.9), and Ornish −3.3 (7.3). Participants were asked to rate their dietary adherence throughout the trial. As shown

Box 4

The Obesity Guidelines[5] subjected 18 diets to systematic evidence review and found no one diet superior in producing weight loss. There are multiple pathways to dietary success.

Box 5

Dietary adherence is the most powerful predictor of weight loss success, a relationship shown in every diet study assessing dietary adherence.

in **Fig. 1**, as adherence increases, weight loss increases, for every type of diet.[34] **Fig. 3** depicts the participants ratings of their dietary adherence on a scale of 1 to 10 over the year. As shown in **Fig. 3**, for each diet, adherence decreased over time[34] (**Box 4**).

In a 2014 meta-analysis of 48 diet trials that include more than 7286 participants, adherence was the best predictor of weight loss success, leading to the conclusion that any diet a patient will adhere to lose weight is the best.[35] As a result, most recommendations are that the patient should play a role in choosing the diet they will undertake. Interestingly, dietary choice has not been proved to make patients more successful in their weight loss efforts. A systematic review and meta-analysis of 12 interventions in 9 studies where patients were able to choose the diet or were assigned the diet did not show any weight loss benefit for choice.[36]

Precision Nutrition and Nutrigenomics

In September 2020 the NIH approved the concept for a new program: "Nutrition for Precision Health, Powered by the All of Us Research Program." Nutrition for Precision Health seeks to move away from population-based nutrition advice. This is good news for research funding in the area. However, there are no successful examples of dietary counseling based on genetic profiles. The missing piece of the nutrigenomics puzzle is evidence that counseling to genetic clues derived from earlier studies produces more weight loss when the information is used prospectively.

Physical Activity

As shown in **Table 1**, the physical activity recommendations for the gold-standard interventions were based primarily on number of minutes of weekly moderate physical activity (usually brisk walking or cycling), from 150 to 225 minutes per week. It is important to meet patients where they are at with their current activity levels and consider starting a regimen of walking (10 minutes 3 times weekly) and gradually building from there, because this goal was the strategy in these studies.

Many individuals believe that physical activity alone can result in clinically meaningful weight loss. However, this idea has been debunked. Jakicic[36] showed that groups of nondieting individuals who engaged in either 150 or 300 minutes of weekly activity both lost less than 2% of initial weight at 6 months. Thus, during the initiation of weight loss the emphasis in behavioral programs is primarily on diet. However, for maintenance, higher amounts of physical activity are particularly effective for promoting long-term weight loss. For example, successful long-term weight loss maintainers report high levels of physical activity averaging 2827 kcal/week in energy expenditure[37] (**Boxes 5** and **6**).

Resistance training has the potential to enhance long-term weight loss by stimulating increased levels of fat oxidation both during and acutely following the exercise session.[38,39] In addition, resistance training may have a positive effect on weight loss

Box 6

Many individual believe that exercise without dieting can easily produce weight loss. This is not true.

Box 7

Behaviors that promote long-term maintenance of lost weight include frequent weighing (even daily, large amounts of aerobic physical activity and regular healthy meals [including breakfast]).

maintenance by preserving or increasing fat-free mass and thereby enhancing metabolic rate.[40] A growing body of evidence supports the potential of resistance training to be a weight loss maintenance tool. For example, Hunter and colleagues determined that resistance training (3 d/wk) enhanced weight loss maintenance following a very-low-calorie diet (800 kcal/d).[41] The proposed mechanism through which resistance training enhanced weight loss maintenance was by preserving fat-free mass, which helped to avert the decline in resting energy expenditure typically seen following calorie restricted weigh loss.[41]

Maintenance of Lost Weight

As noted in other chapters, the body has compensatory mechanisms that defend fat mass, making weight loss difficult. After weight loss, compensatory biological and physiologic mechanisms drive an increase in food intake and decrease in energy expenditure. These mechanisms result in weight regain. In addition, with the current physical and social environment supporting unhealthy dietary practices and sedentary behavior, it is not surprising that initial success in lifestyle programs is commonly followed by a return to pretreatment patterns of eating and physical activity.[41] Indeed, the potency of environmental challenges often initiates a behavioral "cascade" wherein initial lapses in the maintenance of behavioral changes undermine the individual's confidence in their self-management skills and thereby lead to poor long-term adherence and the eventual abandonment of the entire behavior change effort for many individuals.[42,43]

The National Weight Control Registry provides an opportunity to study the habits of successful long-term weight loss maintainers. The strategies that were reported most often in sustaining lost weight are regular self-monitoring of body weight, with 36% reporting weighing once daily and 79% reported weighing once weekly, and high levels of physical activity.[37,44,45] Approximately 75% of these individuals reported expending greater than 1000 kcal/wk (or walking > 10 miles/wk), 54% expending greater than 2000 kcal/wk, and 35% expending greater than 3000 kcal/wk through various forms of physical activity. The dietary pattern is regular, healthy meals, including breakfast[46] (**Box 7**).

SUMMARY

Lifestyle intervention can help some, but not all patients, succeed with long-term weight loss. Those successful patients can achieve health benefits. For patients who do not succeed with lifestyle intervention, intensification is indicated, and medical device and surgical approaches can be implemented to aid in weight loss. Lifestyle intervention is a critical component of *all* obesity care, be it with use of medications, devices, or surgery.

CLINICS CARE POINTS

- A fundamental tenet of all guidance and recommendations for obesity management is that lifestyle intervention—changing behaviors around diet and physical activity—is foundational; that is, all other approaches with medications, devices, and surgery rest on lifestyle changes.

- The weight loss effort begins with setting a goal and timeline; a goal of 10% weight loss from baseline in 6 to 12 months is clinically meaningful.
- Referral to community-based or commercial lifestyle intervention delivery is acceptable, provided programs are guidelines-based and have evidence to support their efficacy and safety.
- There are multiple pathways to dietary success. The best predictor of dietary success is adherence.
- During the initiation of weight loss, the diet receives the most attention; for maintenance of lost weight, physical activity seems most important.
- Not all patients will succeed with lifestyle intervention despite their best efforts; adding medical or surgical therapy is appropriate when patients need the health benefits of weight loss.

DISCLOSURE

Dr D.H. Ryan has served as a Scientific Advisor or Consultant to the following companies: Altimmune, Amgen, Boehringer Ingelheim, Calibrate, Carmot, Epitomee, Gila Therapeutics, IFA Celtic, Lilly, Novo Nordisk, real appeal (United Health), Scientific Intake, Wondr Health, Xeno Bioscience, Ysopia, and Zealand. She has served on the Speakers' Bureau for Novo Nordisk; has received stock options in Epitomee, Calibrate, Roman, and Scientific Intake; and has served on a Data Safety Monitoring Board for setmelanotide, a medication marketed by Rhythm.

FUNDING TEXT

Dr Ryan was partly supported by the grant from the National Institute of General Medical Sciences (U54GM104940) of the National Institutes of Health.

REFERENCES

1. Santos I, Sniehotta FF, Marques MM, et al. Prevalence of personal weight control attempts in adults: a systematic review and meta-analysis. Obes Rev 2017;18(1): 32–50.
2. Malik VS, Willet WC, Hu FB. Nearly a decade on — trends, risk factors and policy implications in global obesity. Nat Rev Endocrinol 2020;16:615–6.
3. Hales CM, Carroll MD, Fryar CD, et al. Prevalence of obesity and severe obesity among adults: United States, 2017–2018. NCHS Data Brief, no 360. Hyattsville, MD: National Center for Health Statistics; 2020.
4. US Preventive Services Task Force. Behavioral Weight Loss Interventions to Prevent Obesity-Related Morbidity and Mortality in Adults: US Preventive Services Task Force Recommendation Statement. JAMA 2018;320(11):1163–71.
5. Jensen MD, Ryan DH, Donato KA, et al. Guidelines (2013) for managing overweight and obesity in adults. Obesity 2014;22(S2):S1–410.
6. Garvey WT, Mechanick JI, Brett EM, et al. American Association of Clinical Endocrinologists and American College of Endocrinology Comprehensive Clinical Practice Guidelines for Medical Care of Patients with Obesity-Executive Summary. Endocr Pract 2016;22(7):842–84.

7. Apovian CM, Aronne LJ, Bessesen DH, et al. Pharmacologic Management of obesity: An Endocrine Society clinical practice guideline. J Clin Endocrinol Metab 2015;100(2):342–62.
8. Mechanick JI, Apovian C, Brethauer S, et al. Clinical practice guidelines for the perioperative nutrition, metabolic, and nonsurgical support of patients undergoing bariatric procedures - 2019 update: cosponsored by American Association of Clinical Endocrinologists/American College of Endocrinology, The Obesity Society, American Society for Metabolic & Bariatric Surgery, Obesity Medicine Association, and American Society of Anesthesiologists - *Executive summary.* Endocr Pract 2019;25(12):1346–59.
9. Hall KD. What is the required energy deficit per unit weight loss? Int J Obes 2008; 32(3):573–6.
10. Harris JA, Benedict FG. A biometric study of basal metabolism in man. Proc Natl Acad Sci 1919;4:370–3.
11. Mifflin MD, Jeor ST, Hill LA, et al. A new predictive equation for resting energy expenditure in healthy individuals. Am J Clin Nutr 1990;51:241–7.
12. FAO/WHO/UNU. Energy and protein requirements. Geneva: World Health Organisation; 1985.
13. The Diabetes Prevention Program. Design and methods for a clinical trial in the prevention of type 2 diabetes. Diabetes Care 1999;22:623–34.
14. The Diabetes Prevention Program (DPP). description of lifestyle intervention. Diabetes Care 2002;25:2165–71.
15. Knowler WC, Barrett-Connor E, Fowler SE, et al. Reduction in the incidence of type 2 diabetes with lifestyle intervention or metformin. N Engl J Med 2002;346: 393–403.
16. Ryan DH, Espeland MA, Foster GD, et al. Look AHEAD (Action for Health in Diabetes): design and methods for a clinical trial of weight loss for the prevention of cardiovascular disease in type 2 diabetes. Control Clin Trials 2003;24:610–28.
17. The Look AHEAD Research Group. Cardiovascular Effects of intensive lifestyle intervention in type 2 diabetes. N Engl J Med 2013;369:145–54.
18. Pi-Sunyer X, Blackburn G, Brancati FL, et al. Reduction in weight and cardiovascular disease risk factors in individuals with type 2 diabetes: one-year results of the look AHEAD trial. Diabetes Care 2007;30:1374–83.
19. Wing R, the Look AHEAD Research Group. Does lifestyle intervention improve health of adults with overweight/obesity and type 2 diabetes: findings from the Look AHEAD randomized trial. Obesity 2021;29(8):1246–58.
20. Katzmarzyk PT, Martin CK, Newton RL, et al. Weight loss in underserved patients — a cluster-randomized trial. N Engl J Med 2020;383:909–18.
21. Katzmarzyk PT, Martin CK, Newton RL Jr, et al. Promoting Successful Weight Loss in Primary Care in Louisiana (PROPEL): Rationale, design and baseline characteristics. Contemp Clin Trials 2018;67:1–10.
22. Befort CA, VanWormer JJ, Desouza C, et al. Effect of behavioral therapy with in-clinic or telephone group visits vs in- clinic individual visits on weight loss among patients with obesity in rural clinical practice: a randomized clinical trial. JAMA 2021;325:363–72.
23. Befort CA, VanWormer JJ, DeSouza C, et al. Protocol for the rural engagement in primary care for optimizing weight reduction (RE-POWER) Trial: Comparing three obesity treatment models in rural primary care. Contemp Clin Trials 2016;47: 304–14.

24. Katzmarzyk PT, Apolzan JW, Gajewski B, et al. Weight loss in primary care: A pooled analysis of two pragmatic cluster-randomized trials. Obesity 2021; 29(12):2044–54.
25. Centers for Medicaid and Medicare Services. Decision memo for intensive behavioral therapy for obesity (CAG-00423N). Cited August 5, 2022. http://www.cms.gov/medicare-coverage-database/details/nca-decision-memo.aspx?&NcaName=Intensive%20Behavioral%20Therapy%20for%20Obesity&bc=ACAAAAAAIAAA&NCAId=253.
26. Carvajal R, Wadden TA, Tsai AG, et al. Managing obesity in primary care practice: a narrative review. Ann NY Acad Sci 2013;1281:191–206.
27. Armstrong MJ, Mottershead TA, Ronksley PE, et al. Motivational interviewing to improve weight loss in overweight and/or obese patients: a systematic review and meta-analysis of randomized controlled trials. Obes Rev 2011;12(9):709–23.
28. https://blog.marketresearch.com/u.s.-weight-loss-market-shrinks-by-25-in-2020-with-pandemic-but-rebounds-in-2021#:~:text=Market%20size%3A%20The%20value%20of,up%2024%25%20to%20%2472.6%20billion Accessed 8/7/2022.
29. Laudenslager M, Chaudhry ZW, Rajagopal S, et al. Commercial Weight Loss Programs in the Management of Obesity: an Update. Curr Obes Rep 2021;10(2):90–9.
30. Key National DPP Milestones Available at https://www.cdc.gov/diabetes/prevention/milestones.html Accessed August 7, 2022.
31. Program Eligibility Available at https://www.cdc.gov/diabetes/prevention/program-eligibility.html Accessed on August 7, 2022.
32. Program Location Available at https://www.cdc.gov/diabetes/prevention/find-a-program.html Accessed August 7, 2022.
33. 2021 Food & Health Survey. 19 May 2021. https://foodinsight.org/2021-food-health-survey/
34. Dansinger ML, Gleason JA, Griffith JL, et al. Comparison of the Atkins, Ornish, Weight Watchers, and Zone diets for weight loss and heart disease risk reduction: a randomized trial. JAMA 2005;293(1):43–53.
35. Johnston BC, Kanters S, Bandayrel K, et al. Comparison of Weight Loss Among Named Diet Programs in Overweight and Obese Adults: A Meta-analysis. JAMA 2014;312(9):923–33.
36. Jakicic JM, Otto AD, Lang W, et al. The effect of physical activity on 18-month weight change in overweight adults. Obesity 2011;19(1):100–9.
37. Ogden L, Phelan S, Thomas J, et al. Dietary habits and weight maintenance success in high vs low exercisers in the National Weight Control Registry. J Phys Act Health 2014;11:1540–8.
38. Moghetti P, Bacchi E, Brangani C, et al. Metabolic Effects of Exercise. Front Horm Res 2016;47:44–57.
39. Petridou A, Siopi A, Mougios V. Exercise in the management of obesity. Metabolism 2019;92:163–9.
40. Hunter GR, Byrne NM, Sirikul B, et al. Resistance training conserves fat-free mass and resting energy expenditure following weight loss. Obesity 2008;16:1045–51.
41. McEvedy SM, Sullivan-Mort G, McLean SA, et al. Ineffectiveness of commercial weight-loss programs for achieving modest but meaningful weight loss: Systematic review and meta-analysis. J Health Psychol 2017;22:1614–27.
42. Elfhag K, Rossner S. Who succeeds in maintaining weight loss? A conceptual review of factors associated with weight loss maintenance and weight regain. Obes Rev 2005;6:67–85.

43. Jeffery RW, French SA, Schmid TL. Attributions for dietary failures: problems reported by participants in the Hypertension Prevention Trial. Health Psychol 1990;9:315–29.
44. Butryn ML, Phelan S, Hill JO, et al. Consistent self-monitoring of weight: a key component of successful weight loss maintenance. Obesity 2007;15:3091–6.
45. Catenacci VA, Odgen L, Phelan S, et al. Dietary habits and weight maintenance success in high versus low exercisers in the National Weight Control Registry. J Phys Act Health 2014;11:1540–8.
46. Wyatt HR, Grunwald GK, Mosca CL, et al. Long-term weight loss and breakfast in subjects in the National Weight Control Registry. Obes Res 2002;10:78–82.

The Effective Use of Anti-obesity Medications

Sarah H. Schmitz, MD*, Louis J. Aronne, MD, FTOS, DABOM

KEYWORDS

- Obesity pharmacotherapy • Treatment of obesity • Anti-obesity medications
- GLP-1 receptor agonists • Off-label prescribing • Combination therapy

KEY POINTS

- Treating obesity requires an individualized approach, matching each patient with the treatment best suited for them.
- Medications should be tested in sequence and may need to be used in combination for optimal results.
- Prescribing off-label generic medications is one strategy to expand access to obesity treatment.

INTRODUCTION

Obesity is undertreated; 46% of US adults meet criteria for anti-obesity medication (AOM) however, only 0.8% of eligible adults reported using AOMs in the past 30 days in combined samples from the National Health and Nutrition Examination Survey 2015 to 2016 and 2017 to 2018. A greater proportion of current AOM users previously tried lifestyle modifications compared with nonusers.[1] Pharmacotherapy for the management of obesity is indicated in adults with a body mass index (BMI) greater than or equal to 30 kg/m^2 or a BMI greater than or equal to 27 kg/m^2 with at least 1 weight-related comorbidity as an adjunct to lifestyle modifications. While a reduced-calorie diet and increased physical activity have been shown to reduce weight and lower cardiometabolic risk, they are not sufficient for maintaining long-term weight maintenance in most patients. Long-term maintenance is difficult given weight loss results in an increase in appetite and a decrease in energy expenditure.[2] AOMs can overcome the biological compensatory mechanisms that drive weight regain.[3] There are 6 FDA-approved AOMs for long-term use, 3 approved for short-term use, and 1 device that functions as a medication.

Selecting an AOM should be individualized to the patient taking into consideration their unique challenges with weight loss, their goals, the presence of comorbidities,

Division of Endocrinology, Diabetes & Metabolism, New York-Presbyterian Hospital/ Weill Cornell Medical College, Comprehensive Weight Control Center, 1305 York Avenue, 4th Floor, New York, NY 10021, USA
* Corresponding author.
E-mail address: hls9007@med.cornell.edu

Gastroenterol Clin N Am 52 (2023) 661–680
https://doi.org/10.1016/j.gtc.2023.08.003

medication contraindications, and drug-drug interactions. Once a medication is started, the patient should be assessed regularly, ideally monthly at the onset, to assess for efficacy and side effects. If the AOM is not tolerable or efficacious, it should be discontinued and another medication should be trialed. If the medication is effective but the patient reaches a weight loss plateau (often defined as no weight loss for over 1 month), consider increasing the dose of the medication or adding an additional agent targeting a different pathway. Medication efficacy should be re-evaluated at each appointment and behavioral interventions should be reinforced. Weight maintenance requires long-term treatment with regular follow-up.

EXPECTED WEIGHT LOSS WITH ANTI-OBESITY MEDICATIONS VERSUS ALTERNATIVE OBESITY TREATMENTS

Modest weight loss of 5% to 10% has been associated with improvements in blood pressure, cholesterol, and glycemic control.[4] Behavioral interventions have shown weight loss of up to 7% to 8% with 80% of weight being regained over 10 years.[5] In phase 3 clinical trials, AOMs have consistently produced greater weight loss than placebo when combined with lifestyle modifications. While the efficacy of first-generation AOMs ranged from 5% to 10% weight loss, the newer AOMs can produce 10% to 15% weight loss. There are several medications in the pipeline with efficacy approaching surgical weight loss. See **Fig. 1** for the efficacy of current and pending AOMs, sleeve gastrectomy, and behavioral interventions.

ON-LABEL ANTI-OBESITY MEDICATIONS

Phentermine

Phentermine is a sympathomimetic amine that is thought to suppress appetite and thereby decrease food intake. See **Fig. 2** demonstrating the mechanism of action of phentermine and all AOMs discussed in this article. It was approved for short-term treatment of obesity (less than 3 months) in 1959 and it is the most commonly prescribed AOM in the United States.[14,15] Phentermine is only approved for short-term use because safety data came from a short-term study and at the time of its approval there was a lack of understanding of the chronic nature of obesity. Phentermine is also approved in pediatric patients aged 16 to 18 years old.[16]

Efficacy

In a 28-week randomized controlled trial (RCT), monotherapy with phentermine 15 mg daily produced a 6 kg weight loss and 46% of the participants achieved 5% or more

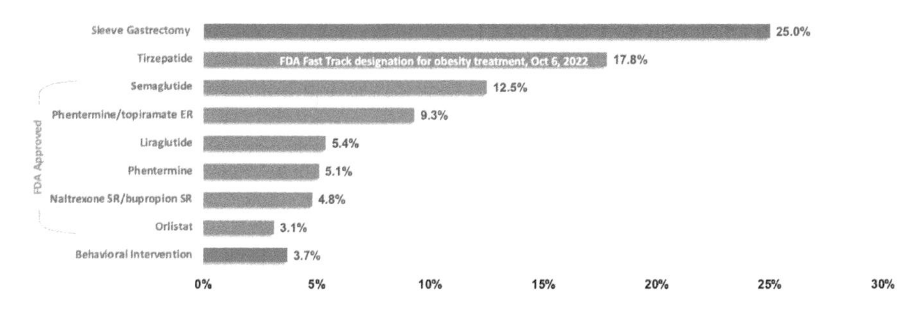

Fig. 1. Efficacy of obesity treatments. (*Data from* Refs.[5–13])

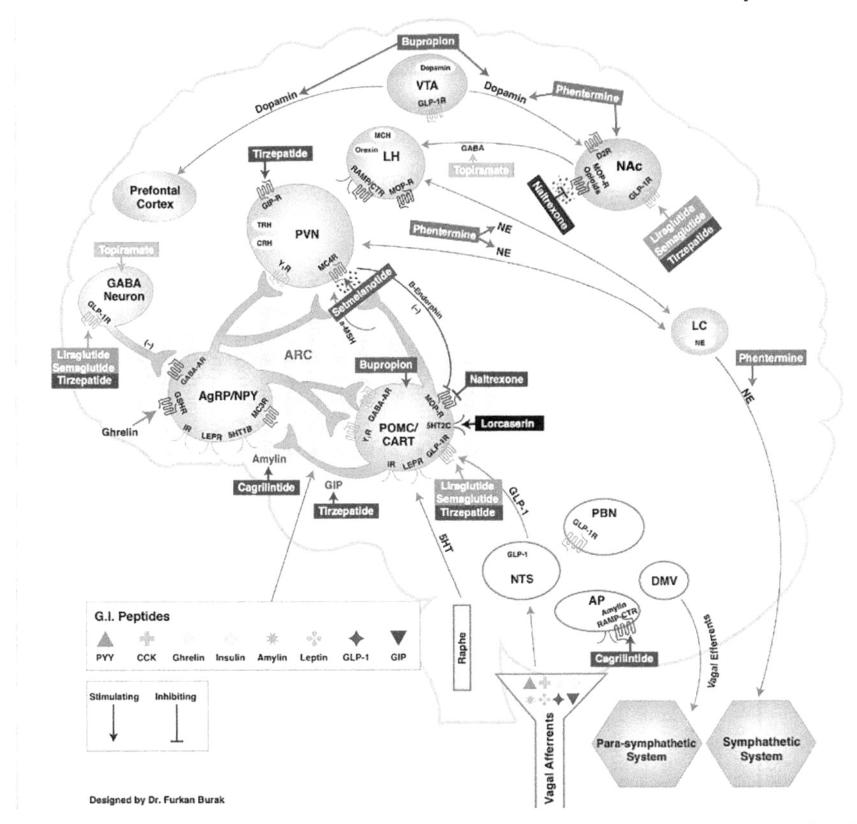

Fig. 2. Mechanism of drug action in obesity. (Burak MF, Istfan NW, Apovian CM. Mechanisms of Drug action in Obesity. Handbook of Obesity, Volume 2: Clinical Applications. Fifth edition. Eds. George A. Bray and Claude Bouchard., Copyright © 2023 by CRC Press. Reproduced by permission of Taylor & Francis Group.)

weight loss.[6] In a 36-week study, 64 patients were randomized to phentermine 30 mg daily, phentermine 30 mg intermittently (4 weeks on, 4 weeks off), or placebo. Participants in both phentermine groups lost about 13% of their initial body weight while participants in the placebo group lost 5%.[17] A 2019 retrospective cohort study reported that patients with a BMI greater or equal to 27 kg/m^2 who took phentermine consistently for over 12 months lost significantly more weight than those who took the medication for less than 3 months (−7.4% vs −0.2%), and the incidence of the composite cardiovascular disease outcome or death was rare (0.3%, 41 events) with no significant difference between groups.[18]

Prescribing and administration

- See **Table 1** for dosing and safety information
- Phentermine is a schedule IV-controlled substance.
- Avoid evening administration as it can lead to insomnia.
- While it is approved for short-term use, many providers prescribe phentermine for long-term use off-label for continued weight management.

Consider in

- Patients who would benefit from appetite suppression.

Table 1
On-label anti-obesity medications

Generic Name	Brand Name	Dosing	Side Effects	Safety
Phentermine	Lomaira Adipex	8 mg tablet daily – TID 37.5 mg tablet half tab daily – BID or 1 tab daily	• Elevation in blood pressure and pulse • Anxiety • Insomnia • Dry mouth • Constipation • Irritability • Palpitations	Contraindicated in: • Cardiovascular disease • Uncontrolled hypertension • Hyperthyroidism • Glaucoma • History of substance use disorder • Pregnancy or nursing • Use of monoamine oxidase inhibitors within the last 14 d • Estimated glomerular filtration rate(eGFR) <15 Caution in • Anxiety • Pulmonary hypertension • eGFR of 15–29 (reduce dose)
Orlistat	Xenical Alli	One 120 mg capsule TID with meals One 60 mg capsule TID with meals	• Fatty or oily stool • Oil spotting • Fecal urgency • Rare cases of severe liver injury with hepatocellular necrosis or acute liver failure have been reported	Contraindicated in • Pregnancy • Chronic malabsorption • Cholestasis May interact with • Cyclosporine • Warfarin • Amiodarone • Antiepileptics • Antiretrovirals • Levothyroxine (administer 4 h apart)

Phentermine/topiramate	Qsymia	3.75 mg/23 mg daily (starting dose) 7.5 mg/46 mg daily (lowest treatment dose) 11.25 mg/69 mg daily (titration dose) 15 mg/92 mg daily (maximum treatment dose)	• Elevation in blood pressure and pulse • Dry mouth • Constipation • Paresthesias • Nausea • Vomiting • Insomnia • Dizziness • Anxiety • Irritability • Impaired cognition • Disturbances in attention	Contraindicated in • Cardiovascular disease • Uncontrolled hypertension • Hyperthyroidism • Pregnancy • Glaucoma • Use of monoamine oxidase inhibitors within the last 14 d Caution in • Anxiety • History of kidney stones
Bupropion/naltrexone	Contrave	1 tablet (90 mg/8 mg) daily for week 1 Increase by 1 tablet weekly until daily maintenance dose of 2 tablets twice a day is achieved at week 4	• Nausea • Vomiting • Constipation • Diarrhea • Elevated blood pressure and pulse • Insomnia • Dry mouth • Elevated liver enzymes and hepatotoxicity have been reported in patients taking naltrexone	Contraindicated in • Uncontrolled hypertension • Use of opioid agonists or partial agonists • History of seizures • Bulimia or anorexia nervosa • Pregnancy • Use of monoamine oxidase inhibitors within the last 14 d Caution in • Anxiety May interact with • Can increase serum concentrations of drugs metabolized by CYP2D6 • May effect concentration of digoxin

(*continued on next page*)

Table 1
(continued)

Generic Name	Brand Name	Dosing	Side Effects	Safety
Liraglutide 3.0	Saxenda	Inject 0.6 mg subcutaneously daily for 1 week. In weekly intervals, increase the dose by 0.6 mg until a dose of 3.0 mg daily is reached.	• Nausea • Vomiting • Abdominal pain • Diarrhea • Constipation • Dyspepsia • Fatigue • Acute pancreatitis • Acute cholecystitis • Acute kidney injury secondary to dehydration • Hypoglycemia (especially in those with type 2 diabetes taking concomitant insulin or insulin secretagogues) • Elevated heart rate	Contraindicated in • Personal or family history of medullary thyroid cancer • Personal or family history of multiple endocrine neoplasia syndrome type 2 (MEN 2) • Pregnancy (discontinue at least 2 mo before pregnancy) • History of idiopathic pancreatitis • Should not be used in combination with other glucagon-like-peptide-1 (GLP-1) receptor agonists Caution in • History of diabetic retinopathy • Uncontrolled diabetes (?) • May impact absorption of oral medications
Semaglutide 2.4	Wegovy	Inject 0.25 mg subcutaneously weekly. Increase every 4 wk to 0.5 mg, 1.0 mg, 1.7 mg, and 2.4 mg sequentially.		
Gelesis100	Plenity	3 oral capsules with 500 mL of water 20–30 min before lunch and dinner	• Diarrhea • Abdominal distention • Infrequent bowel movements • Flatulence • Dyspepsia	Contraindicated in • Gastric motility issues • Esophageal anatomic abnormalities • Pregnancy Caution in • Active gastroesophageal reflux disease • Gastric ulcers

Adapted from Schmitz, S., Tchang, B.G. & Shukla, A.P. Obesity Pharmacotherapy: a Review of Current Practices and Future Directions. Curr Treat Options Gastro 21, 27–47 (2023). https://doi.org/10.1007/s11938-023-00409-1.

Other sympathomimetic amines

Phendimetrazine and diethylpropion are also approved for short-term treatment of obesity and are less commonly used than phentermine. They are schedule IV and III controlled substances, respectively.

Orlistat

Orlistat is a gastrointestinal lipase inhibitor that decreases the absorption of dietary fat. It was Food and Drug Administration (FDA) approved for the treatment of obesity in 1999 for adults and in 2003 for adolescents aged 12 to 16. A lower dose is approved for over-the-counter use under the trade name Alli for patients with a BMI of 25 kg/m^2 and above.

Efficacy

In the XENical in the prevention of Diabetes in Obese Subjects (XENDOS) trial, 3305 patients with obesity at risk for type 2 diabetes were randomized to lifestyle changes plus orlistat 120 mg 3 times daily versus placebo. At the end of the 4-year trial, mean weight loss was significantly greater with orlistat versus placebo (5.8 kg vs 3.0 kg).[19] In a meta-analysis of 16 orlistat trials of 1 to 4 years duration with a total of 10,631 participants, orlistat reduced weight by 2.9 kg or 2.9% more than placebo and increased the absolute percentage of participants achieving 5% and 10% weight loss thresholds by 21% and 12%, respectively.[20]

Prescribing and administration

See **Table 1** for dosing and safety information.

- Orlistat may reduce the absorption of fat-soluble vitamins; therefore, patients should be advised to take a multivitamin.[20]
- Orlistat is not commonly used in clinical practice given the modest weight loss effect in combination with the side effect profile.

Consider in

- Patients with chronic constipation including medication-induced constipation.

Phentermine/Topiramate Extended Release

Phentermine/topiramate extended release (ER) is a fixed-dose combination medication approved in 2012 for the long-term treatment of obesity. Phentermine is a sympathomimetic amine and topiramate, which is FDA approved for the treatment of epilepsy and migraine prophylaxis, has been shown to reduce body weight by decreasing caloric intake and promoting taste aversion.[21]

Efficacy

The 56-week phase 3 Controlled-Release Phentermine/Topiramate in Severely Obese Adults (EQUIP) trial enrolled 1267 participants with obesity and reported 9.3% placebo-subtracted weight loss in the maximum treatment dose group (15/92 mg).[7] The 1-year Collaborative, National Quality and Efficacy Registry (CONQUER) trial randomized 2487 patients with a BMI of 27 to 45 kg/m^2 and 2 or more comorbidities (hyperlipidemia, hypertension, diabetes or prediabetes, or abdominal obesity) to a mid-dose treatment dose (7.5/46 mg), a maximum treatment dose (15/92 mg), or placebo and reported 6.6% and 8.6% placebo-subtracted weight loss in the mid and maximum dose arms, respectively.[15] In a 2-year extension of the CONQUER trial (SEQUEL), mean placebo-subtracted weight loss was 7.5% in the mid-dose group and 8.7% in the maximum-dose group.[22]

In a 2022 meta-analysis that included a total of 49,810 participants and 143 trials of AOMs, phentermine/topiramate ER was the most effective oral drug for weight loss.[23]

Prescribing and administration

- See **Table 1** for dosing and safety information.
- Phentermine is a schedule IV-controlled substance.
- Topiramate is teratogenic; therefore, women of childbearing potential should have a pregnancy test prior to starting the medication and need to use effective contraception while taking the medication.
- Providers should enroll in a Risk Evaluation and Mitigation Strategy (REMS) to inform women of reproductive potential about the increased risk of cleft lip/palate in fetuses exposed to topiramate in the first trimester of pregnancy.

Consider in

- Patients who would benefit from appetite suppression and enhanced satiety.
- Patients who have migraines.

Bupropion Sustained Release/Naltrexone Sustained Release

Bupropion, a norepinephrine and dopamine reuptake inhibitor, and naltrexone, an opioid receptor antagonist, are FDA approved as a fixed-dose combination pill for long-term weight management. Bupropion stimulates hypothalamic proopiomelanocortin (POMC) neurons with downstream effects of reduced food intake and increased energy expenditure.[24] Naltrexone blocks POMC autoinhibition, augmenting the effects of bupropion.[25]

Efficacy

In the Contrave Obesity Research (COR)-1 trial, a 56-week double-blind RCT, mean weight loss was 6.1% in the bupropion/naltrexone 360 mg/32 mg group versus 1.3% in the placebo group. About half of the participants (48%) lost at least 5% of their body weight in the treatment group versus 16% in the placebo group.[8] Adding intensive behavioral therapy to bupropion/naltrexone produces greater weight loss (9.3% with treatment vs 5.2% with placebo).[26]

Prescribing and administration

See **Table 1** for dosing and safety information.

Consider in

- Patients who would benefit from appetite suppression or decreased cravings.
- Patients who are trying to quit smoking.
- Patients who are trying to reduce alcohol intake.

Liraglutide 3.0

Liraglutide is a glucagon-like-peptide-1 (GLP-1) receptor agonist FDA approved for obesity treatment in adults and children 12 years and older with obesity and a body weight above 60 kg. GLP-1 is an incretin hormone that acts in the gastrointestinal tract to reduce gastric emptying thereby increasing satiation. The GLP-1 receptor is also present in the brain where it is involved in appetite regulation.[27]

Efficacy

Liraglutide was studied in three 56-week randomized double-blind placebo-controlled trials. In Satiety and Clinical Adiposity—Liraglutide Evidence (SCALE) Obesity and Prediabetes, (n = 3731) mean weight loss was 8% with liraglutide 3.0 mg/d versus 2.6% in the placebo group. In the SCALE maintenance study, (n = 422) participants who lost at least 5% of their initial body weight on a low-calorie diet were randomized to liraglutide 3.0 mg/d vs. placebo for 56 weeks. Mean initial weight loss was 6.0%.

Those in the treatment group lost an additional 6.2% compared to 0.2% in the placebo group.[28]

In patients with type 2 diabetes, liraglutide 1.8 mg/d has been shown to reduce major adverse cardiovascular events.[29] Cardiovascular outcomes data in patients without type 2 diabetes are not available.

Prescribing and administration

See **Table 1** for dosing and safety information.

- If results are adequate or the patient has side effects during dose titration continue or reduce the dose as clinically appropriate.

Consider in

- Patients who would benefit from appetite suppression and increased satiety.
- Patients with type 2 diabetes.
- Patients with prediabetes or insulin resistance.

Semaglutide 2.4

Semaglutide is a long-acting GLP-1 receptor agonist FDA approved for chronic weight management in adults and pediatric patients aged 12 years and older with a BMI at greater or equal to the 95th percentile standardized for age and sex. Semaglutide slows gastric emptying, thereby reducing energy intake, in addition to directly acting on the brain to reduce food reward and cravings.[30] It is considered the most effective AOM available given it produced the largest percentage reduction in body weight in clinical trials.

Efficacy

The Semaglutide Treatment Effect in People with obesity (STEP) trials were double-blind, randomized, multicenter studies conducted over 68 weeks. They evaluated the efficacy of semaglutide 2.4 mg once weekly on weight reduction in patients with overweight or obesity, with and without type 2 diabetes. In STEP 1 (n = 1961), there was a 14.9% reduction in body weight in the semaglutide 2.4 mg group versus a 2.4% reduction in the placebo group. This trial was conducted in adults with overweight or obesity without type 2 diabetes.[9] In STEP 2 (n = 1210) which included participants with overweight or obesity and type 2 diabetes, average placebo-subtracted weight loss was 6.2% in the treatment group.[31]

In the STEP 4 trial, (n = 902) subjects were randomized to continue treatment with semaglutide 2.4 mg weekly or switch to placebo for 48 weeks after a 20-week run-in period on semaglutide. Mean weight loss was 10.6% among the 803 patients who completed the run-in period. Subjects who continued on semaglutide lost an additional 7.9% of their body weight while those who switched to placebo gained 6.8% of their body weight.[32]

STEP 5 (n = 304) was a 2-year trial that assessed the safety and effectiveness of semaglutide 2.4 mg weekly versus placebo in addition to lifestyle interventions for long-term weight loss. Mean change in body weight was −15.2% in the treatment group vs −2.6% in the placebo group.[33]

STEP 8 (n = 338) was a 68-week randomized open-label trial that compared semaglutide 2.4 mg weekly versus liraglutide 3 mg daily. Weight loss was 15.8% in the semaglutide group compared to 6.4% in the liraglutide group. Treatment discontinuation occurred more often in the liraglutide group (27.6% vs 13.5%).[34]

In patients with type 2 diabetes, semaglutide 1.0 mg weekly has been shown to improve cardiovascular outcomes.[35] A cardiovascular outcome trial (CVOT) for semaglutide 2.4 mg in patients without type 2 diabetes is underway (SELECT, NCT03574597).

Prescribing and administration
See **Table 1** for dosing and safety information.

- Discontinue at least 2 months before a planned pregnancy.

Consider in

- Patients who would benefit from appetite suppression and increased satiety.
- Patients with type 2 diabetes.
- Patients with prediabetes or insulin resistance.

SETMELANOTIDE

Setmelanotide is FDA approved for the treatment of monogenic obesity and will be discussed in another section.

Gelesis100

Gelesis100 was FDA approved for weight management in 2019 for those with a BMI of 25 to 40 kg/m^2 regardless of comorbidities. The capsules in combination with water form a hydrogel matrix which occupies about one-quarter of the average stomach volume, creating a sensation of fullness. The matrix is later digested and eliminated in the stool. Gelesis100 is considered a medical device given it has no systemic effects.[36]

Efficacy
In the Gelesis Loss of Weight (GLOW) RCT, which included participants with a BMI of 27 kg/m^2 and above, mean weight loss at 6 months was 6.4% in the gelesis100 group versus 4.4% in the placebo group in.[37]

Prescribing and administration
See **Table 1** for dosing and safety information.
Consider in

- Patients with a BMI in the 25 to 27 kg/m^2 range.
- Patients who prefer a non-systemically absorbed product.

Cost Considerations

Economic sustainability needs to be considered when prescribing AOMs given obesity is a chronic disease and medications should be used long term. Currently, Medicare does not cover AOMs and in many states Medicaid does not cover these medications as well. The monthly out-of-pocket cost for on-label AOMs without insurance coverage ranges from $6 to 8 for phentermine to $1400 for semaglutide.[38] Prescribing off-label generic medications is one strategy to expand access to obesity treatment. In 2022, the Institute for Clinical and Economic Review published an evidence report on the comparative clinical effectiveness and cost of phentermine/topiramate (Qsymia), bupropion/naltrexone (Contrave), liraglutide (Saxenda), and semaglutide (Wegovy) for weight management. Phentermine/topiramate was the most cost-effective option and if prescribed generically could be cost saving.[39]

Off-Label Anti-obesity Medications

Metformin
Metformin is a diabetes medication that has been available in some countries since the 1950s. It is used off-label for the treatment of obesity given it promotes weight loss through multiple potential mechanisms including increasing leptin sensitivity,[40]

increasing serum levels of GLP-1 peptide,[41] increasing serum levels of anorexigenic GDF-15 peptide,[42] and improving insulin sensitivity.[43]

Efficacy

In the Diabetes Prevention Program Outcomes Study, 28.5% of the participants were considered "responders" to metformin as they achieved greater than or equal to 5% weight loss at 1 year. Among responders, average weight loss was maintained at 6% to 8% over 15 years.[5] A retrospective cohort study compiled 6-month and 12-month weight loss outcomes in patients with or without type 2 diabetes or prediabetes on metformin monotherapy at doses of 1500 to 2000 mg per day. Average weight loss was similar between the euglycemic and type 2 diabetes/prediabetes groups at both 6 and 12 months (6 months: 6.5 [6.0%] vs 6.5 [6.1%] $P = .97$; 12 months: 7.4 [6.2%] vs 7.3 [7.7%], $P = .92$). The proportion of patients who achieved at least 5% weight loss was greater than 50% in both groups.[44]

Metformin is also efficacious for the treatment of antipsychotic-induced weight gain.[45]

Prescribing and administration

Initiate treatment at 500 mg daily, preferably with the extended release version to improve tolerability. Increase the dose to 1000 mg per day in 1 to 2 weeks as needed and tolerated. Can gradually increase to 2000 mg per day as maximum dose.

Recommend taking metformin with food to improve tolerability.

Consider in

- Patients with type 2 diabetes.
- Patient with prediabetes or insulin resistance.
- Patients with polycystic ovary syndrome (PCOS).
- Patients with antipsychotic-induced weight gain.
- Patients with perimenopausal weight gain.

Topiramate

Topiramate is FDA approved for the treatment of epilepsy and migraine prevention. Topiramate is used off label for weight management and is particularly helpful in patients with binge eating disorder, night eating, or recurrent thoughts about food.

Efficacy

A 6-month RCT showed that topiramate is effective for weight loss; those in the topiramate 96 mg/day, 192 mg/day, and 256 mg/day groups lost 7.0%, 9.1%, and 9.7% of their baseline body weight, respectively, while those in the placebo group lost 1.7%. There were associated improvements in blood pressure and glucose tolerance.[21]

Prescribing and administration

Start with 25 mg before dinner, can increase by 25 to 50 mg/day weekly. Range 25 to 200 mg daily.

Topiramate decreases contraceptive efficacy and increases breakthrough bleeding, especially at doses greater than 200 mg/day.

Patients on doses of 100 mg/day or more require gradual dose taper prior to discontinuation to prevent seizures.

Consider in

- Patients who have migraine headaches.
- Patients with binge eating behaviors.
- Patients with night eating.

- Patients with recurrent thoughts about food.

Bupropion

Bupropion is FDA approved for major depressive disorder and smoking cessation. Bupropion is a preferred agent for depression given it can cause weight loss as a side effective whereas most other antidepressants can cause weight gain when used long-term.[46] It is used off label for weight management.

Efficacy

A 48-week randomized trial reported 7.2% weight loss in the bupropion sustained release (SR) 300 mg group and 10.1% in the bupropion SR 400 mg group versus 5.0% in the placebo group. This trial also included lifestyle modifications. The percentage of participants who lost at least 5% of their initial body weight was 46%, 59%, and 83% for placebo, bupropion SR 300 mg, and 400 mg, respectively.[47]

Prescribing and administration

Bupropion is available in immediate release (IR), sustained release (SR), and extended release (XR) versions. Start with SR 100 mg or XL 150 mg daily in the morning. The dose can be increased to SR 100 mg twice a day or XL 300 mg daily in 1 to 2 weeks as needed. IR dosing is not commonly used given the need for 3 times daily dosing.

Consider in

- Patients who would benefit from decreased cravings.
- Patients who are trying to quit smoking.
- Patients with depression.

Naltrexone

Naltrexone is FDA approved for the treatment of alcohol use disorder and prevention of relapse in opioid use disorder. Naltrexone is used off label for weight management and is often considered in patients with food cravings and recurrent thoughts on food.

Efficacy

Although no clinical trials have been done with naltrexone alone for weight loss, smaller studies have found associations between naltrexone and both reduced food intake and reduced reward properties of food.[48,49]

Prescribing and administration

Naltrexone is available as a 50 mg pill. Recommend starting with one-fourth tablet (12.5 mg). After 1 to 2 weeks can increase to half tablet (25 mg). Range 12.5 to 50 mg daily.

Consider in

- Patients who would benefit from decreased cravings.
- Patients with binge eating.
- Patients with concomitant alcohol use disorder.
- Patients interested in reducing alcohol consumption.

Zonisamide

Zonisamide, an FDA approved antiseizure drug, is also used off label for weight management.

Efficacy

In a 1-year randomized-controlled study in patients with obesity, the mean percentage change in body weight was −6.8% in the zonisamide 400 mg group versus −3.7% in the placebo group. A total of 55% of patients in the zonisamide 400 mg group lost at least 5% of their body weight versus 31% in the placebo group.[50]

Prescribing and administration

Start with 25 mg once daily. Can increase by 25 mg every 1 to 2 weeks as needed and tolerated.

Consider in

- Patients with binge eating.
- Patients with emotional eating.
- Patients with night eating.

Oral Semaglutide

The oral form of semaglutide is FDA approved for the management of type 2 diabetes. It is used off label for weight management.

Efficacy

In the Randomized Clinical Trial of the Efficacy and Safety of Oral Semaglutide Monotherapy in Comparison With Placebo in Patients With Type 2 Diabetes (PIONEER 1) trial, oral semaglutide 14 mg/d resulted in a mean reduction in body weight of 4.1 kg compared to placebo in individuals with type 2 diabetes and obesity.[51] In the Efficacy and Safety of Oral Semaglutide 50 mg Once Daily in Subjects With Overweight or Obesity (OASIS-1) trial, a phase 3 68-week RCT, oral semaglutide 50 mg daily produced 17.4% weight loss versus 1.8% weight loss in the placebo group in patients without type 2 diabetes.[52] The authors anticipate approval of oral semaglutide for weight management given the OASIS-1 data.

Prescribing and administration

Start with 3 mg daily. Can increase the dose every month to 7 mg and finally to a maximum dose of 14 mg as tolerated.

The medication must be taken with about 4 ounces of water on an empty stomach 30 minutes prior to food or medication.

Consider in

- Patients with type 2 diabetes.
- Patients with prediabetes or insulin resistance.
- Patients with PCOS.

Sodium-Glucose Transport-2 inhibitors

Sodium-glucose transport-2 inhibitors (SGLT-2) inhibitors are FDA approved for the treatment of type 2 diabetes. These medications are proposed to cause weight loss via glucosuria-induced osmotic diuresis and calorie loss.[53]

Efficacy

In a 24-week clinical trial, patients with type 2 diabetes and obesity on metformin lost 2.08 kg with the addition of dapaglifozin 10 mg daily versus those on metformin alone.[53] A meta-analysis of 116 RCTs investigating the weight reduction effects of SGLT inhibitors was published in early 2022. In the cohort of 98,497 patients with and without diabetes, a mean weight reduction of 1.79 kg was seen in patients on any SGLT drug compared to placebo. Mean BMI changes were −0.71 kg/m^2 compared to placebo. Dual SGLT1/SLGT2 inhibitors were associated with a significantly greater reduction in weight relative to SGLT2 inhibitors.

These medications are not currently approved in the United States but are available in Europe.[54]

Safety

The most common side effects of SGLT-2 inhibitors include dehydration, urinary tract infections, and genital mycotic infections. They are contraindicated in patients with an estimated glomerular filtration rate (eGFR) less than 30 and patients on dialysis.[55–58]

Prescribing and administration

Varies by SGLT-2 inhibitor.

Consider in

- Patients with type 2 diabetes or prediabetes.
- Patients with nephropathy.
- Patients with cardiovascular disease.
- Patients with heart failure.

Tirzepatide

Tirzepatide is a glucose-dependent insulinotropic polypeptide (GIP) receptor and GLP-1 receptor agonist currently approved for the treatment of type 2 diabetes. The exact mechanism of GIP as it relates to weight loss is unknown but it is thought to enhance the anorexigenic effect and tolerability of the GLP-1 agonist component.

Efficacy

In the Efficacy and Safety of Tirzepatide Once Weekly in Participants without Type 2 Diabetes Who Have Obesity or are Overweight with Weight Related Comorbidities (SURMOUNT-1) trial, tirzepatide was studied for weight management in people with overweight or obesity without diabetes (n = 2539). The 72-week phase 3 RCT randomized participants to tirzepatide 5 mg, 10 mg, or 15 mg or placebo. Mean weight loss in the 15 mg weekly group was 20.9% versus 3.1% in the placebo group. Almost all (91%) participants in the tirzepatide 15 mg weekly group had a weight reduction of 5% or more versus 35% of those in the placebo group.[10] In SURMOUNT-2, tirzepatide 10 mg and 15 mg were studied for weight management in participants with overweight or obesity and type 2 diabetes. Those in the tirzepatide 10 mg group lost 13.4% of their body weight and those in the 15 mg group lost 15.7% of their body weight compared to a 3.3% reduction in the placebo group.[59] The authors anticipate approval for tirzepatide for weight management given the SURMOUNT data.

Safety

Tirzepatide has a similar side effect profile to the GLP-1 receptor agonists. Side effects include nausea, abdominal pain, diarrhea, constipation, reflux, vomiting, and increased heart rate. Hypoglycemia can occur when used in combination with insulin or insulin secretagogues.

Prescribing and administration

Administered via weekly subcutaneous injection at doses of 2.5 mg, 5 mg, 7.5 mg, 10 mg, 12.5 mg, and 15 mg. Start with 2.5 mg weekly and increase the dose every 4 weeks as needed and tolerated.

Consider in

- Patients with type 2 diabetes.
- Patients with prediabetes or insulin resistance.
- Patients with inadequate weight loss with semaglutide 2.4 mg.

Combination Anti-obesity Regimens

Two or more AOMs are often needed to achieve and maintain clinically significant long-term weight loss.[3] In a retrospective review of patients treated at a tertiary obesity management center, the use of 2 or more AOMs was associated with significantly greater likelihood of greater than or equal to 5% weight loss over 2 years.[60]

Current evidence for combination therapies is summarized as follows.

- Bupropion 200 mg/d in combination with zonisamide 400 mg/d resulted in 7.2 kg weight loss vs. 2.9 kg with zonisamide alone.[61]
- Canagliflozin 300 mg/d in combination with metformin 2000 mg/d,[62] phentermine 15 mg/d,[63] or liraglutide 1.8 mg/d[64] has consistently resulted in more weight loss than the respective monotherapies in short-term trials (<1 year).
- Empagliflozin 12.5 mg BID plus metformin 1000 mg BID demonstrated superior short-term weight loss relative to the individual components.[65]
- An RCT evaluating the effect of liraglutide 3.0 mg plus phentermine in adults following 1 year of treatment with liraglutide alone found no additional weight loss with the combination.[66]

DISCUSSION

Obesity is a complex, chronic, relapsing disease; therefore, successful treatment requires the use of all treatment modalities available. As the number of AOMs continues to grow, providers have the unique challenge of determining which medication is the most appropriate for a given patient. When selecting an AOM, many variables need to be considered including the presence of comorbidities, medication contraindications, side effect profile, patient preference, and cost and insurance coverage. For example, in a patient with obesity and type 2 diabetes, a GLP-1 receptor agonist should be considered provided there are no contraindications. If the patient prefers to avoid injectable medications, oral semaglutide could be considered. If insurance does not cover this medication, an SGLT-2 inhibitor or metformin could be initiated. Regular monitoring and follow-up with a provider is crucial to ensure safe and effective use of AOMs. It is important to remember that there is wide patient-to-patient variability in response to a given AOM. If a medication is not effective, other medications should be trialed. Additive therapies are often necessary to counteract metabolic adaptations to weight loss. Cost and insurance coverage are important issues to consider given treatment is lifelong. The AOM pipeline includes several promising agents with efficacy rivaling surgical weight loss.

CLINICS CARE POINTS

- Pharmacologic therapy is indicated in patients with a BMI greater or equal to 30 kg/m^2 or a BMI $\geq$ 27 kg/m^2 with at least 1 weight-related comorbidity.[67]
- Pharmacotherapy should be prescribed in combination with a comprehensive lifestyle management plan.
- Medication selection should be individualized to the patient to optimize benefits versus risks.
- Pharmacotherapy should treat both weight and comorbidities.
- Medication doses should be individualized to the patient with the lowest effective dose being used to obtain an adequate response.

- Given there is wide heterogeneity in the causes of obesity, there is also patient-to-patient variability in the response to individual AOMs.
- If a patient has not lost at least 4% to 5% of baseline body weight after 12 to 16 weeks at the maintenance dose of an AOM, consider discontinuing the medication given clinically meaningful weight loss is unlikely to be achieved with continued treatment.
- Consider using combinations of AOMs to overcome the biological compensatory mechanisms that occur with weight loss.[3]
- Off-label prescribing is often necessary to overcome barriers to care including difficulties with insurance coverage.
- Pharmacotherapy should be prescribed with the intention of long-term (for life) use given obesity is a chronic disease. If an effective AOM is discontinued, weight regain is likely.[32]

DISCLOSURE

S.H. Schmitz reports no disclosures. L.J. Aronne reports receiving consulting fees from/and serving on advisory boards for Allurion, Altimmune, Atria, Gelesis, Jamieson Wellness, Janssen Pharmaceuticals, Jazz Pharmaceuticals, Novo Nordisk, Pfizer, Optum, Eli Lilly, Senda Biosciences and Versanis; receiving research funding from Allurion, AstraZeneca, United Kingdom, Gelesis, Janssen Pharmaceuticals, United States, Novo Nordisk and Eli Lilly; having equity interests in Allurion, ERX Pharmaceuticals, Gelesis, Intellihealth, Jamieson Wellness and Myos Corp; and serving on a board of directors for ERX Pharmaceuticals, Intellihealth and Jamieson Wellness.

REFERENCES

1. MacEwan J, Kan H, Chiu K, et al. Antiobesity Medication Use Among Overweight and Obese Adults in the United States: 2015-2018. Endocr Pract 2021;27(11): 1139–48.
2. Rosenbaum M, Hirsch J, Gallagher DA, et al. Long-term persistence of adaptive thermogenesis in subjects who have maintained a reduced body weight. Am J Clin Nutr 2008;88(4):906–12.
3. Aronne LJ, Hall KD, Jakicic J, et al. Describing the Weight-Reduced State: Physiology, Behavior, and Interventions. Obesity 2021;29(Suppl 1):S9–24.
4. Ryan DH, Yockey SR. Weight Loss and Improvement in Comorbidity: Differences at 5%, 10%, 15%, and Over. Curr Obes Rep 2017;6(2):187–94.
5. Apolzan JW, Venditti EM, Edelstein SL, et al, Diabetes Prevention Program Research Group. Long-Term Weight Loss With Metformin or Lifestyle Intervention in the Diabetes Prevention Program (DPP) Outcomes Study (DPPOS). Ann Intern Med 2019;170(10):682–90.
6. Aronne LJ, Wadden TA, Peterson C, et al. Evaluation of phentermine and topiramate versus phentermine/topiramate extended-release in obese adults. Obesity 2013;21(11):2163–71.
7. Allison DB, Gadde KM, Garvey WT, et al. Controlled-release phentermine/topiramate in severely obese adults: a randomized controlled trial (EQUIP). Obesity 2012;20(2):330–42.
8. Greenway FL, Fujioka K, Plodkowski RA, et al, COR-I Study Group. Effect of naltrexone plus bupropion on weight loss in overweight and obese adults (COR-I): a multicentre, randomised, double-blind, placebo-controlled, phase 3 trial. Lancet 2010;376(9741):595–605.

9. Wilding JPH, Batterham RL, Calanna S, et al, STEP 1 Study Group. Once-Weekly Semaglutide in Adults with Overweight or Obesity. N Engl J Med 2021;384(11): 989–1002.
10. Jastreboff AM, Aronne LJ, Ahmad NN, et al, SURMOUNT-1 Investigators. Tirzepatide Once Weekly for the Treatment of Obesity. N Engl J Med 2022;387(3): 205–16.
11. Mechanick JI, Apovian C, Brethauer S, et al. Clinical practice guidelines for the perioperative nutrition, metabolic, and nonsurgical support of patients undergoing bariatric procedures - 2019 update: cosponsored by American Association of Clinical Endocrinologists/American College of Endocrinology, The Obesity Society. American Society for Metabolic & Bariatric Surgery, Obesity Medicine Association, and American Society of Anesthesiologists. Surg Obes Relat Dis. 2020;16(2):175–247.
12. Pi-Sunyer X, Astrup A, Fujioka K, et al. A Randomized, Controlled Trial of 3.0 mg of Liraglutide in Weight Management. N Engl J Med 2015;373(1):11–22.
13. Finer N, James WP, Kopelman PG, et al. One-year treatment of obesity: a randomized, double-blind, placebo-controlled, multicentre study of orlistat, a gastrointestinal lipase inhibitor. Int J Obes Relat Metab Disord 2000;24(3):306–13.
14. Thomas CE, Mauer EA, Shukla AP, et al. Low adoption of weight loss medications: A comparison of prescribing patterns of antiobesity pharmacotherapies and SGLT2s. Obesity 2016;24(9):1955–61.
15. Gadde KM, Allison DB, Ryan DH, et al. Effects of low-dose, controlled-release, phentermine plus topiramate combination on weight and associated comorbidities in overweight and obese adults (CONQUER): a randomised, placebo-controlled, phase 3 trial. Lancet 2011;377(9774):1341–52.
16. Singhal V, Sella AC, Malhotra S. Pharmacotherapy in pediatric obesity: current evidence and landscape. Curr Opin Endocrinol Diabetes Obes 2021;28(1): 55–63.
17. Munro JF, MacCuish AC, Wilson EM, et al. Comparison of continuous and intermittent anorectic therapy in obesity. Br Med J 1968;1(5588):352–4.
18. Lewis KH, Fischer H, Ard J, et al. Safety and Effectiveness of Longer-Term Phentermine Use: Clinical Outcomes from an Electronic Health Record Cohort. Obesity 2019;27(4):591–602.
19. Torgerson JS, Hauptman J, Boldrin MN, et al. XENical in the prevention of diabetes in obese subjects (XENDOS) study: a randomized study of orlistat as an adjunct to lifestyle changes for the prevention of type 2 diabetes in obese patients. Diabetes Care 2004;27(1):155–61.
20. Rucker D, Padwal R, Li SK, et al. Long term pharmacotherapy for obesity and overweight: updated meta-analysis. BMJ 2007;335(7631):1194–9.
21. Wilding J, Van Gaal L, Rissanen A, et al. A randomized double-blind placebo-controlled study of the long-term efficacy and safety of topiramate in the treatment of obese subjects. Int J Obes Relat Metab Disord 2004;28(11):1399–410.
22. Garvey WT, Ryan DH, Look M, et al. Two-year sustained weight loss and metabolic benefits with controlled-release phentermine/topiramate in obese and overweight adults (SEQUEL): a randomized, placebo-controlled, phase 3 extension study. Am J Clin Nutr 2012;95(2):297–308.
23. Shi Q, Wang Y, Hao Q, et al. Pharmacotherapy for adults with overweight and obesity: a systematic review and network meta-analysis of randomised controlled trials. Lancet 2022;399(10321):259–69.
24. Greenway FL, Whitehouse MJ, Guttadauria M, et al. Rational design of a combination medication for the treatment of obesity. Obesity 2009;17(1):30–9.

25. Billes SK, Sinnayah P, Cowley MA. Naltrexone/bupropion for obesity: an investigational combination pharmacotherapy for weight loss. Pharmacol Res 2014; 84:1–11.
26. Wadden TA, Foreyt JP, Foster GD, et al. Weight loss with naltrexone SR/bupropion SR combination therapy as an adjunct to behavior modification: the COR-BMOD trial. Obesity 2011;19(1):110–20.
27. Drucker DJ. GLP-1 physiology informs the pharmacotherapy of obesity. Mol Metab 2022;57:101351.
28. Wadden T, Hollander P, Klein S, et al. Weight maintenance and additional weight loss with liraglutide after low-calorie-diet-induced weight loss: The SCALE Maintenance randomized study. Int J Obes 2013;37:1443–51.
29. Marso SP, Daniels GH, Brown-Frandsen K, et al. Liraglutide and Cardiovascular Outcomes in Type 2 Diabetes. N Engl J Med 2016;375(4):311–22.
30. Knudsen LB, Lau J. The Discovery and Development of Liraglutide and Semaglutide. Front Endocrinol 2019;10:155.
31. Davies M, Færch L, Jeppesen OK, et al, STEP 2 Study Group. Semaglutide 2·4 mg once a week in adults with overweight or obesity, and type 2 diabetes (STEP 2): a randomised, double-blind, double-dummy, placebo-controlled, phase 3 trial. Lancet 2021;397(10278):971–84.
32. Rubino D, Abrahamsson N, Davies M, et al, STEP 4 Investigators. Effect of Continued Weekly Subcutaneous Semaglutide vs Placebo on Weight Loss Maintenance in Adults With Overweight or Obesity: The STEP 4 Randomized Clinical Trial. JAMA 2021;325(14):1414–25.
33. Garvey WT, Batterham RL, Bhatta M, et al, STEP 5 Study Group. Two-year effects of semaglutide in adults with overweight or obesity: the STEP 5 trial. Nat Med 2022;28(10):2083–91.
34. Rubino DM, Greenway FL, Khalid U, et al, STEP 8 Investigators. Effect of Weekly Subcutaneous Semaglutide vs Daily Liraglutide on Body Weight in Adults With Overweight or Obesity Without Diabetes: The STEP 8 Randomized Clinical Trial. JAMA 2022;327(2):138–50.
35. Marso SP, Bain SC, Consoli A, et al, SUSTAIN-6 Investigators. Semaglutide and Cardiovascular Outcomes in Patients with Type 2 Diabetes. N Engl J Med 2016;375(19):1834–44.
36. Plenity (Gelesis100) [package insert]. Boston, MA: Gelesis, Inc.; 2019.
37. Greenway FL, Aronne LJ, Raben A, et al. A Randomized, Double-Blind, Placebo-Controlled Study of Gelesis100: A Novel Nonsystemic Oral Hydrogel for Weight Loss. Obesity 2019;27(2):205–16.
38. Prescription prices CpilGcOAfhwgc.
39. Atlas SJ, Kim K, Beinfeld M, et al. *Medications for Obesity Management: Effectiveness and Value; Final Evidence Report*, 20, 2022, Institute for Clinical and Economic Review. Available at: https://icer.org/wp-content/uploads/2022/03/ICER_Obesity_Final_Evidence_Report_and_Meeting_Summary_102022.pdf.
40. Kim YW, Kim JY, Park YH, et al. Metformin restores leptin sensitivity in high-fat-fed obese rats with leptin resistance. Diabetes 2006;55(3):716–24.
41. Preiss D, Dawed A, Welsh P, et al, DIRECT consortium group. Sustained influence of metformin therapy on circulating glucagon-like peptide-1 levels in individuals with and without type 2 diabetes (CAMERA). Diabetes Obes Metabol 2017; 19(3):356–63.
42. Coll AP, Chen M, Taskar P, et al. GDF15 mediates the effects of metformin on body weight and energy balance. Nature 2020;578(2295):444–8.

43. Yerevanian A, Soukas AA. Metformin: Mechanisms in Human Obesity and Weight Loss. Current Obesity Reports 2019;8(2):156–64.
44. Chukir T, Mandel L, Tchang BG, et al. Metformin-induced weight loss in patients with or without type 2 diabetes/prediabetes: A retrospective cohort study. Obes Res Clin Pract 2021;15(1):64–8.
45. Wu RR, Zhao JP, Jin H, et al. Lifestyle intervention and metformin for treatment of antipsychotic-induced weight gain: a randomized controlled trial. JAMA 2008; 299(2):185–93.
46. Gafoor R, Booth HP, Gulliford MC. Antidepressant utilisation and incidence of weight gain during 10 years' follow-up: population based cohort study. BMJ 2018;361:k1951.
47. Anderson JW, Greenway FL, Fujioka K, et al. Bupropion SR enhances weight loss: a 48-week double-blind, placebo- controlled trial. Obes Res 2002;10(7):633–41.
48. Langleben DD, Busch EL, O'Brien CP, et al. Depot naltrexone decreases rewarding properties of sugar in patients with opioid dependence. Psychopharmacology (Berl) 2012;220(3):559–64.
49. Spiegel TA, Stunkard AJ, Shrager EE, et al. Effect of naltrexone on food intake, hunger, and satiety in obese men. Physiol Behav 1987;40(2):135–41.
50. Gadde KM, Kopping MF, Wagner HR, et al. Zonisamide for weight reduction in obese adults: a 1-year randomized controlled trial. Arch Intern Med 2012; 172(20):1557–64.
51. Aroda VR, Rosenstock J, Terauchi Y, et al, PIONEER 1 Investigators. PIONEER 1: Randomized Clinical Trial of the Efficacy and Safety of Oral Semaglutide Monotherapy in Comparison With Placebo in Patients With Type 2 Diabetes. Diabetes Care 2019;42(9):1724–32.
52. Knop FK, Aroda VR, do Vale RD, et al. Oral semaglutide 50 mg taken once per day in adults with overweight or obesity (OASIS 1): a randomised, double-blind, placebo-controlled, phase 3 trial. Lancet 2023;402(10403):705–19.
53. Bolinder J, Ö Ljunggren, Kullberg J, et al. Effects of dapagliflozin on body weight, total fat mass, and regional adipose tissue distribution in patients with type 2 diabetes mellitus with inadequate glycemic control on metformin. J Clin Endocrinol Metab 2012;97(3):1020–31.
54. Cheong AJY, Teo YN, Teo YH, et al. SGLT inhibitors on weight and body mass: A meta-analysis of 116 randomized-controlled trials. Obesity 2022;30(1):117–28.
55. Farxiga (dapagliflozin) [package insert]. Wilmington, DE: AstraZeneca Pharmaceuticals; 2014.
56. Invokana (canagliflozin) [package insert]. Titusville, NJ: Janssen Pharmaceuticals; 2013.
57. Jardiance (empagliflozin) [package insert]. Indianapolis, IN: Eli Lilly and Company; 2014.
58. Steglatro (ertugliflozin) [package insert]. Whitehouse Station, NJ: Merck & Co; 2017.
59. Garvey WT, Frias JP, Jastreboff AM, et al. Tirzepatide once weekly for the treatment of obesity in people with type 2 diabetes (SURMOUNT-2): a double-blind, randomised, multicentre, placebo-controlled, phase 3 trial. Lancet 2023; 402(10402):613–26.
60. Tchang BG, Aras M, Wu A, et al. Long-term weight loss maintenance with obesity pharmacotherapy: A retrospective cohort study. Obesity Science Practice 2022; 8(3):320–7.

61. Gadde KM, Yonish GM, Foust MS, et al. Combination therapy of zonisamide and bupropion for weight reduction in obese women: a preliminary, randomized, open-label study. J Clin Psychiatr 2007;68(8):1226–9.
62. Rosenstock J, Chuck L, González-Ortiz M, et al. Initial Combination Therapy With Canagliflozin Plus Metformin Versus Each Component as Monotherapy for Drug-Naïve Type 2 Diabetes. Diabetes Care 2016;39(3):353–62.
63. Hollander P, Bays HE, Rosenstock J, et al. Coadministration of Canagliflozin and Phentermine for Weight Management in Overweight and Obese Individuals Without Diabetes: A Randomized Clinical Trial. Diabetes Care 2017;40(5):632–9.
64. Ali AM, Martinez R, Al-Jobori H, et al. Combination Therapy With Canagliflozin Plus Liraglutide Exerts Additive Effect on Weight Loss, but Not on HbA. Diabetes Care 2020;43(6):1234–41.
65. Hadjadj S, Rosenstock J, Meinicke T, et al. Initial Combination of Empagliflozin and Metformin in Patients With Type 2 Diabetes. Diabetes Care 2016;39(10):1718–28.
66. Tronieri JS, Wadden TA, Walsh OA, et al. Effects of liraglutide plus phentermine in adults with obesity following 1 year of treatment by liraglutide alone: A randomized placebo-controlled pilot trial. Metabolism 2019;96:83–91.
67. Jensen MD, Ryan DH, Apovian CM, et al, American College of Cardiology/American Heart Association Task Force on Practice Guidelines, Obesity Society. 2013 AHA/ACC/TOS guideline for the management of overweight and obesity in adults: a report of the American College of Cardiology/American Heart Association Task Force on Practice Guidelines and The Obesity Society. Circulation 2014;129(25 Suppl 2):S102–38.

Emerging Endoscopic Interventions in Bariatric Surgery

Joshua S. Winder, MD[a], John H. Rodriguez, MD[b,*]

KEYWORDS

• Endoscopy • Bariatric endoscopy • Endoscopic sleeve gastroplasty
• Gastric aspiration • Incisionless magnetic anastomosis • Endoluminal barrier sleeve

KEY POINTS

- Various endoscopic techniques have been developed to treat obesity and metabolic disease.
- These techniques vary widely from implantable devices to gastric remodeling.
- Endoscopic strategies for treatment include both malabsorptive and restrictive models.
- These interventions generally are well tolerated and provide improvement in both weight management and metabolic disease.

INTRODUCTION

Obesity continues to be a major health care concern, and, despite great efforts, it continues to affect a growing number of people in all age groups worldwide.[1] Bariatric surgery has been shown to be an effective tool for weight loss and improvement of weight-related comorbidities and has an acceptable risk profile.[2] Despite the proven efficacy of metabolic surgery, only a small number of individuals have access to high-quality surgical care. This trend likely is multifactorial, including issues with cost, access, and patient preference. Although bariatric surgery is relatively safe, it is not without risk, with reported rates of morbidity ranging from 3% to 20% and mortality rates ranging from 0.1% to 0.5%.[3,4] Endoscopic options to treat obesity are compelling options for many reasons. Endoscopy generally is less invasive. Depending on the technique or device used, endoscopy may be less expensive. Endoscopic therapies can be used as a bridge to further therapies for patients whose comorbidities may limit their surgical options. Conversely, many patients may not qualify for bariatric surgery (body mass index [BMI] >35 kg/m^2 with comorbidities or BMI >40 kg/m^2) but still be

[a] Division of Minimally Invasive and Bariatric Surgery, Penn State Milton S. Hershey Medical Center, Hershey, PA, USA; [b] Department of General Surgery, Cleveland Clinic Abu Dhabi, Al Maryah Island, Abu Dhabi P.O. Box 112412, United Arab Emirates
* Corresponding author.
E-mail address: rodrigj2@clevelandclinicabudhabi.ae

Gastroenterol Clin N Am 52 (2023) 681–689
https://doi.org/10.1016/j.gtc.2023.09.001
gastro.theclinics.com

may interested or benefit from weight loss. Various techniques in endoscopic interventions in bariatric surgery (EIBSs) have emerged and generally fall into 2 different categories: procedures and devices. This review examines the procedure or device, its efficacy, and any risks or adverse events associated with its use. EIBS devices include intragastric space-occupying devices (discussed elsewhere), gastric aspiration devices, incisionless magnetic anastomotic systems, and endoluminal bypass barrier sleeves. EIBS procedures include primary obesity surgery endoluminal (POSE), endoscopic sleeve gastroplasty (ESG), and duodenal mucosal resurfacing (DMR).

DEVICES

Gastric Aspiration Devices

Aspiration therapy works by inserting a tube, similar to a percutaneous endoscopic gastrostomy tube, and then aspirating a portion of the ingested contents into an external reservoir, which then is disposed of. This lessens the amount of chime, and therefore calories, that then is transmitted downstream for digestion and absorption by the gut. The Aspire Assist system (Aspire Bariatrics, King of Prussia, Pennsylvania) is a Food and Drug Administration (FDA)-approved device that is inserted with a typical pull-technique under endoscopic guidance. After the tract is developed, approximately 1 to 2 weeks post procedure, the external tubing is trimmed short and connected to an external skin port. The Aspire Assist has been approved in the United States for use in patients with BMI between 35 and 55 kg/m^2. Multiple small studies have shown promising results with regards to weight loss using the Aspire Assist device. Noren and colleagues[5] saw a mean percentage of excess weight loss (%EWL) of 54.5% 28.8% at 1 year and BMI dropped from a mean of 39.8 kg/m^2 at inclusion to 32.1 kg/m^2. Forssell and colleagues[6] showed a mean %EWL of 40.8% 19.8% at 6 months in patients with a starting mean BMI of 40.3 kg/m^2. In a 12-month multicenter US trial, 171 patients underwent lifestyle counseling and treatment with the Aspire Assist device or lifestyle counseling alone.[7] The investigators found a significant difference in %EWL and improvement in weight-related comorbidities in the treatment group. The baseline mean BMI for patients treated with the device was 42.2 kg/m^2. The mean %EWL in the treatment group was 37.2% 27.5% compared with 13.0% 17.6% in the control group. Hemoglobin (Hgb)A_{1c} levels decreased to an average of 0.36%, relative to 5.7% at baseline ($P < .0001$). High-density lipoprotein cholesterol increased by 8.1% (P5 .0001), and triglycerides decreased by 9.9% (P5 .02). The most common adverse events reported in the study included peristomal granulation tissue, postoperative abdominal pain, peristomal irritation, nausea, abdominal discomfort, and peristomal bacterial infection. Early removal rate during the first year was 26.1%.

Aspiration therapy benefits from at least 2 mechanisms for weight loss: aspiration of calories and behavior changes. In a pilot study examining the Aspire Assist device, Sullivan and colleagues[8] found that 25% to 30% of calories from a meal were aspirated if performed according to protocol. This means that only 80% of weight loss seen can be attributed to aspiration of the ingested meal. The remaining 20% likely was due to the patient-reported decrease in food intake and food particles that must be small in size (<5 mm) and in a slurry to be removed adequately. This factor requires the patient to chew more thoroughly and ingest adequate amounts of water for the catheter to work, with both of these practices leading to smaller portion sizes.

Incisionless Magnetic Anastomotic Systems

The Incisionless Magnetic Anastomotic System (GI Windows, West Bridgewater, Massachusetts) takes advantage of a dual-path anastomotic enteral bypass, which allows nutrients to follow their normal path through the gastrointestinal (GI) tract or through the bypassing anastomosis created with opposing magnetic discs. In this way, it may be classified as a malabsorptive procedure. The coupling discs are deployed using pediatric colonoscopes in the jejunum and ileum, respectively. Once the magnets are coupled, they create an anastomosis by causing local tissue necrosis and remodeling between the 2 discs. In the first human pilot study of the device, 10 patients with a mean baseline BMI of 41 kg/m^2 underwent combined endoscopic and laparoscopic placement (to ensure proper coupling and limb length).[9] At 12 months, the patients had experienced a 40.2%EWL. Improvement in HgbA$_{1c}$ was 1.9% for diabetic patients and 1.0% for prediabetic patients. Most patients complained of transient nausea and all patients had diarrhea with the procedure, which resolved. Four patients had recurrent diarrhea that responded to diet modification. This device is not yet FDA approved.

ENDOLUMINAL BYPASS BARRIER SLEEVES

Duodenojejunal Bypass Sleeve

The first endoluminal implant used to induce weight loss by malabsorption was the duodenojejunal bypass sleeve (DJBS).[10] The Endo Barrier (GI Dynamics, Lexington, Massachusetts) is a DJBS that is covered with polytetrafluoroethylene, making it impermeable to nutrients. The device is deployed endoscopically within the duodenal bulb with a nitinol anchor that works like a self-expanding metal stent, which is connected to a long sleeve that extends distally approximately 65 cm into the jejunum. The Teflon coated tube transports the ingested food through the duodenum and proximal jejunum without allowing interaction with the mucosa, thus prohibiting absorption. The biliary and pancreatic secretions flow freely down the outside of the tube, eventually mixing with the ingested food further downstream. This system can stay in situ for 3 to 12 months. It currently is approved for use in Europe for patients with type 2 diabetes mellitus and obesity for 12 months. It was approved for use in Europe in 2010, but currently is not approved for use in the United States.

In the first prospective trial of the device, 12 patients with a baseline mean BMI of 43 kg/m^2 had the device implanted for 12 weeks.[11] Mean %EWL was 23.6% at 12 weeks and, of the 4 patients with diabetes included in the study, 3 discontinued their diabetic medications. The average baseline BMI was 43 kg/m^2 and the average ending BMI was 38.7 kg/m^2. Two patients had the device removed prior to the 12 weeks due to abdominal pain, and 2 injuries occurred during removal of the device (an oropharyngeal and esophageal mucosal tear), which did not require further intervention.

In a subsequent human trial of the device, 25 patients with a mean starting BMI of 42 kg/m^2 were randomized to either device implantation or dietary modification for a 12-week period.[12] The investigators reported a 22%EWL for the device group versus 5%EWL for the controls. They did see 3 patients with upper GI bleeds, 1 anchor migration, and 1 stent obstruction.

In the first European trial of the device, 41 patients were randomized to either device implantation or a diet control group[13]; 30 patients were randomized to the device group and 11 to the control group. Of the 30 randomized to the device group, 26 devices were safely implanted and 4 were removed early due to migration, dislocation of the anchor, obstruction, or continuous epigastric pain. Mean %EWL for the device group was 19.0% whereas the control group was 6.9%EWL ($P < .002$). Mean BMI at inclusion for the device group was 48.9 kg/m^2 and mean absolute BMI reduction over the study period was 5.5 kg/m^2; 8 patients of the device group were living with diabetes at baseline and showed improvement in 7 patients during the study period (lower glucose levels, $HgbA_{1c}$, and medication requirements). All patients in the device group reported abdominal pain and nausea for the first week following implantation.

In a 52-week prospective, open-label clinical trial of the DJBS, 22 patients with obesity and type 2 diabetes mellitus were recruited.[14] Their mean BMI at the start of the study was 44.8 kg/m^2. Of the 22 patients, 13 completed the 52-week study period. At the end of 1 year, the investigators noted an impressive reduction in $HgbA_{1c}$ levels (2.1% 0.3%). For those 9 patients who had the stent removed early, reasons for removal included device migration (n 5 3), hemorrhage (n 5 1), abdominal pain (n 5 2), principal investigator request (n 5 2), and discovery of an unrelated malignancy (n 5 1). For those patients who completed the study, the most common device-related adverse events were upper abdominal pain (n 5 11), back pain (n 5 5), nausea (n 5 7), and vomiting (n 5 7).

Gastroduodenal-Jejunal Bypass Sleeve

The gastroduodenal-jejunal bypass sleeve is another form of endoscopic barrier bypass, which is anchored at the gastroesophageal junction using a combined endoscopic/laparoscopic approach (Endo Bypass System [ValenTx, Hopkins, Minnesota]). This device extends distally through the stomach and 120 cm into the small bowel, more closely mimicking traditional Roux-en-Y gastric bypass anatomy.

In the first series of patients with 1 year of implantation of this device, the results seemed favorable. In the study, 13 patients with a mean baseline BMI of 42 kg/m^2 were included. Of the 13 patients enrolled, 10 completed the study period (1 patient did not have the device implanted due to inflammation at the gastroesophageal junction at the time of attempted placement, and 2 patients had the device removed early due to intolerance).[15] Six of the 10 patients who had the device implanted had fully attached and functional devices throughout the study period (the remaining 4 had partial detachment). The mean %EWL was 35.9% for the entire group, but was even higher for patients who had fully attached devices (54%EWL). The Endo Bypass System did not receive FDA approval. It did achieve a CE mark in 2009 which was subsequently withdrawn in 2017.

PROCEDURES

Two main procedures have been developed for gastric body remodeling in an attempt to help restrict the distensibility of the stomach and reduce the amount of food ingested by creating a sensation of early satiety. These procedures are the POSE and the ESG. Both procedures do require a separate endoscopic device to complete the procedure and are considered restrictive.

Primary Obesity Surgery Endoluminal

POSE is accomplished with the Incisionless Operating Platform (USGI Medical, San Clemente, California). This is a stand-alone device with 4 working channels that accommodate tissue graspers, an ultraslim camera, and tissue anchors. It measures approximately 54F and is maneuvered like a typical endoscope. The procedure is accomplished by placing 8 to 10 plicating anchors along a double-ridge configuration to reduce the size and shape of the fundic apex down to the level of the gastroesophageal junction. This reduces the volume of the stomach, limiting the amount that can be ingested, and increases gastric emptying time.

In a prospective case series presented by Lopez-Nava and colleagues,[16] for patients who underwent POSE and were followed-up at 1 year, the mean %EWL was of 44.9% 24.4%. Their mean baseline BMI was 38.0 kg/m^2. In their series of 147 patients, they had no serious short-term or long-term adverse events associated with the procedure.

In a recent, multicenter, randomized, sham-controlled trial, 332 patients were randomized in a 2:1 ratio to the POSE procedure or sham, with both groups receiving low-intensity lifestyle therapy.[17] The baseline mean BMI for patients in the treatment arm was 36.0 kg/m^2. The procedure success rate was 99.5%, and the procedure time was 40.0 minutes 12.9 minutes. After 1 year, the investigators reported a mean %TBWL (total body weight loss) of 4.95 7.04% in active and 1.38 5.58% in sham groups, respectively. Significant adverse events included pain, nausea, vomiting, 1 patient with a hepatic abscess, and 1 patient with extraluminal bleeding.

Endoscopic Sleeve Gastroplasty

ESG is an endoscopic procedure using a device called the OverStitch (Apollo Endosurgery, Austin, Texas). This consists of a cap that is placed on the end of a double-channel therapeutic endoscope. The device has a handle that attaches to the shaft of the endoscope at the instrument channels. The cap consists of a curved needle that, when toggled, swings in and out. One of the working channels is used to pass a shuttle device that helps pass the needle back and forth within the device. By using the shuttle and swinging needle, the operator can take full-thickness bites of the target tissue. The OverStitch allows the endoscopist to make various suturing patterns, including running or interrupted, with absorbable or permanent sutures (**Figs. 1–3**).

Initial techniques performing ESG achieved the desired configuration with 6 to 12 stitches, each placed in a triangular fashion at the anterior wall, greater curvature, and posterior wall. Sharaiha and colleagues[18] described placing a median of 8 sutures in a running fashion by starting in the antrum and moving proximally.[18] This included fundic reduction. They reported that in their series of 23 patients, after 1 year, the mean BMI fell from 34.2 to 29.4 kg/m^2.

In the largest series of patients who underwent ESG, 1000 patients were followed out to 12 months.[19] Their baseline mean BMI was 33.3 kg/m^2 4.5 kg/m^2 and age of 34.4 years 9.5 years. Mean percentages of total weight loss at 6, 12, and 18 months were 13.7% 6.8%, 15.0% 7.7%, and 14.8% 8.5%, respectively. Mean BMI fell from 33.3 to 28.9 kg/m^2 at 18 months. Thirteen of 17 patients with diabetes, all patients with hypertension, and 18 of 32 patients with dyslipidemia were in complete remission by the third month of the study. During the first week following ESG, 92.4% of patients

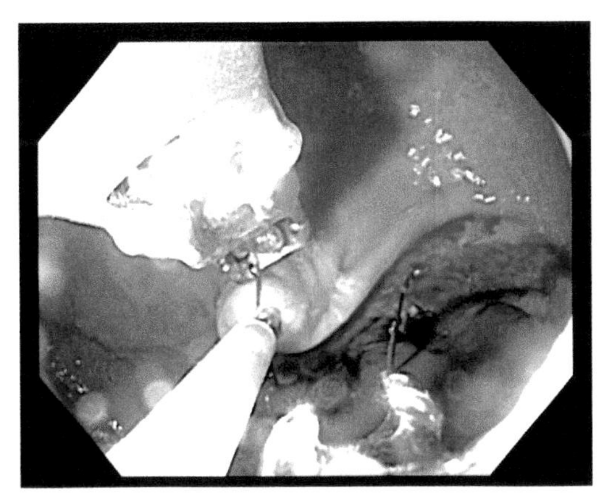

Fig. 1. Endoscopic view of OverStitch (Apollo Endosurgery, Austin, Texas) using tissue helix device to grab and pull full-thickness stomach tissue into the cap allowing for plication during endoscopic sleeve gastroplasty (ESG).

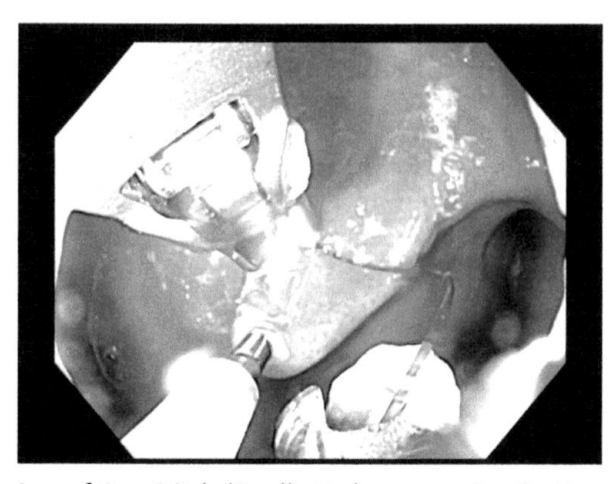

Fig. 2. Endoscopic view of OverStitch (Apollo Endosurgery, Austin, Texas) using tissue helix device to grab and pull full-thickness stomach tissue into the cap allowing for plication during endoscopic sleeve gastroplasty (ESG).

complained of nausea or abdominal pain, which was managed conservatively. Twenty-four patients were readmitted: 8 for severe abdominal pain, 3 of whom ultimately underwent ESG reversal; 7 for post procedure bleeding, 2 of whom required transfusion; 4 for perigastric collections with pleural effusion, with 3 requiring percutaneous drainage; and 5 for post procedure fever with no sequelae.

More recently, the MERIT trial was published in The Lancet. This was the first randomized clinical trial performed at 9 US centers comparing ESG with lifestyle modification (decreased caloric intake and exercise) to lifestyle modification alone. The 9 centers enrolled 209 participants from 2017 to 2019. Patients were followed for 104 weeks with the primary endpoint being %EWL (with goal BMI 25 kg/m^2) at 52 weeks, with secondary endpoints of improvement of obesity-related comorbidities and adverse events from ESG. The baseline characteristics between the groups were similar, with the ESG group being largely female (88%), with a mean BMI of 35.5 kg/m^2. At 52 weeks the mean %EWL was 49.2% for the ESG group compared to 3.2% for the control group ($P < .0001$). With regards to improvement in obesity-related comorbid conditions the

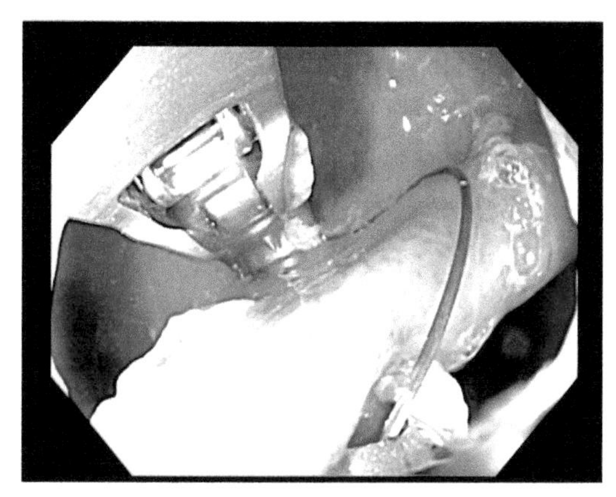

Fig. 3. Endoscopic view of OverStitch (Apollo Endosurgery, Austin, Texas) using tissue helix device to grab and pull full-thickness stomach tissue into the cap allowing for plication during endoscopic sleeve gastroplasty (ESG).

researchers saw statistically significant improvement for the primary ESG group in HbA1c levels, hypertension, HDL and triglyceride levels, metabolic syndrome, as well as liver transaminases, hepatic steatosis index, aspartate transaminase-to-platelets ratio index, and C-reactive protein compared with the control group. Three patients (2%) experienced a procedure-related event including one intraabdominal abscess managed with endoscopic drainage, one upper GI bleed managed conservatively, and one patient with malnutrition requiring ESG reversal.

Duodenal Mucosal Resurfacing

DMR is accomplished by performing a saline lift of the duodenal mucosa distal to the ampulla of Vater to the desired point distally in the duodenum. The lifted mucosa then is hydrothermally ablated using the Revita DMR (Fractyl, Lexington, Massachusetts). The 2-cm long balloon is filled with heated water and the tissue ablated under direct visualization. These steps are repeated along the length of the desired duodenum.

An international multicenter study enrolled 46 patients to undergo DMR.[20] Inclusion criteria included patients with type 2 diabetes mellitus on at least 1 oral hypoglycemic agent with BMI of 20 to 40 kg/m^2. In 37 patients, the procedure was completed successfully (the remaining were unsuccessful due to technical issues), with 36 completing the study protocol. Mean BMI at enrollment was 31.6 kg/m^2. Only 1 significant adverse event (a fever) was reported, which self-resolved. $HgbA_{1c}$ was reduced by 10 mmol/mol 2 mmol/mol (0.9% 0.2%) (mean SD) at 24 weeks ($P < .001$) compared with baseline, and this effect was preserved out to 12 months following DMR. Weight loss was observed for the first 4 weeks post-DMR, which then stabilized. This weight loss did not correlate with the improvement in diabetes control.

SUMMARY

EIBSs include novel devices and techniques that provide various modes of both malabsorptive and constrictive changes to the GI tract. Improvements in weight and metabolic activity have been observed with these techniques, although weight loss and improvement in diabetic control vary between different EIBSs. Most reported studies of these techniques are small case series with short follow-up. More research is needed to fully understand the long-term effect of these modalities and in which populations they would be most beneficial. They do represent an ongoing trend, however, toward less-invasive management strategies that show promising results in this early and exciting period. Currently, of the devices listed, the only FDA approved device is the Aspire Assist which has been approved for patients 22 years of age or older with a BMI of 35 to 55 kg/m^2. When comparing the gastric aspiration device to POSE or ESG, patients must be adherent with a healthy lifestyle and must understand the management of the device for best results. Similarly, to receive the best outcomes from either procedure described here (POSE or ESG), it is recommended that patients follow a healthy lifestyle plan as well as the follow-up protocols on a long-term basis. When considering any of these procedures for your patients, long-term adherence as well as risk/benefit profile should be assessed and discussed in detail.

CLINICS CARE POINTS

- Endoluminal bariatric interventions offer potential treatment for patients with class 1 obesity.

- These procedures and devices have been designed with safety as the top priority to offer patients additional alternatives in the treatment of obesity and related medical conditions.
- Compared to metabolic surgery, these procedures should offer a safer profile despite decreased effectiveness and durability.
- Endoluminal procedures can be utilized as primary intervention, adjuvant therapy, or as a bridge to metabolic surgery in high-risk cases.

DISCLOSURE

J.S. Winder receives consulting fees from Boston Scientific Corp. J.H. Rodriguez has no conflict of interest relevant to this publication. Outside of the scope of this publication, he has received research funding from Pacira Pharmaceuticals and Intuitive Surgical.

REFERENCES

1. Obesity: preventing and managing the global epidemic. Report of a WHO consultation. World Health Organ Tech Rep Ser 2000;894(i-xii):1–253.
2. Schauer PR, Kashyap SR, Wolski K, et al. Bariatric surgery versus intensive medical therapy in obese patients with diabetes. N Engl J Med 2012;366(17):1567–76.
3. Morino M, Toppino M, Forestieri P, et al. Mortality after bariatric surgery: analysis of 13,871 morbidly obese patients from a national registry. Ann Surg 2007;246(6): 1002–7 [discussion 7–9].
4. Buchwald H, Estok R, Fahrbach K, et al. Trends in mortality in bariatric surgery: a systematic review and meta-analysis. Surgery 2007;142(4):621–32 [discussion 32–5].
5. Noren E, Forssell H. Aspiration therapy for obesity; a safe and effective treatment. BMC Obes 2016;3:56.
6. Forssell H, Noren E. A novel endoscopic weight loss therapy using gastric aspiration: results after 6 months. Endoscopy 2015;47(1):68–71.
7. Thompson CC, Abu Dayyeh BK, Kushner R, et al. Percutaneous gastrostomy device for the treatment of class II and class III obesity: results of a randomized controlled trial. Am J Gastroenterol 2017;112(3):447–57.
8. Sullivan S, Stein R, Jonnalagadda S, et al. Aspiration therapy leads to weight loss in obese subjects: a pilot study. Gastroenterology 2013;145(6):1245–12452, e1-5.
9. Machytka E, Buzga M, Zonca P, et al. Partial jejunal diversion using an incisionless magnetic anastomosis system: 1-year interim results in patients with obesity and diabetes. Gastrointest Endosc 2017;86(5):904–12.
10. Patel SR, Mason J, Hakim N. The duodenal-jejunal bypass sleeve (EndoBarrier Gastrointestinal Liner) for weight loss and treatment of type II diabetes. Indian J Surg 2012;74(4):275–7.
11. Rodriguez-Grunert L, Galvao Neto MP, Alamo M, et al. First human experience with endoscopically delivered and retrieved duodenal-jejunal bypass sleeve. Surg Obes Relat Dis 2008;4(1):55–9.
12. Tarnoff M, Rodriguez L, Escalona A, et al. Open label, prospective, randomized controlled trial of an endoscopic duodenal-jejunal bypass sleeve versus low calorie diet for pre-operative weight loss in bariatric surgery. Surg Endosc 2009; 23(3):650–6.
13. Schouten R, Rijs CS, Bouvy ND, et al. A multicenter, randomized efficacy study of the EndoBarrier gastrointestinal liner for presurgical weight loss prior to bariatric surgery. Ann Surg 2010;251(2):236–43.

14. de Moura EG, Martins BC, Lopes GS, et al. Metabolic improvements in obese type 2 diabetes subjects implanted for 1 year with an endoscopically deployed duodenal-jejunal bypass liner. Diabetes Technol Ther 2012;14(2):183–9.
15. Sandler BJ, Rumbaut R, Swain CP, et al. One-year human experience with a novel endoluminal, endoscopic gastric bypass sleeve for morbid obesity. Surg Endosc 2015;29(11):3298–303.
16. Lopez-Nava G, Bautista-Castano I, Jimenez A, et al. The primary obesity surgery endolumenal (POSE) procedure: one-year patient weight loss and safety outcomes. Surg Obes Relat Dis 2015;11(4):861–5.
17. Sullivan S, Swain JM, Woodman G, et al. Randomized sham-controlled trial evaluating efficacy and safety of endoscopic gastric plication for primary obesity: The ESSENTIAL trial. Obesity 2017;25(2):294–301.
18. Sharaiha RZ, Kumta NA, Saumoy M, et al. Endoscopic sleeve gastroplasty significantly reduces body mass index and metabolic complications in obese patients. Clin Gastroenterol Hepatol 2017;15(4):504–10.
19. Alqahtani A, Al-Darwish A, Mahmoud AE, et al. Short-term outcomes of endoscopic sleeve gastroplasty in 1000 consecutive patients. Gastrointest Endosc 2019;89(6):1132–8.
20. van Baar ACG, Holleman F, Crenier L, et al. Endoscopic duodenal mucosal resurfacing for the treatment of type 2 diabetes mellitus: one year results from the first international, open-label, prospective, multicentre study. Gut 2020;69(2):295–303.

Mechanisms of Action of Bariatric Surgery on Body Weight Regulation

Khaled Alabduljabbar, MD[a,b], Efstathios Bonanos, MD[c], Alexander D. Miras, PhD[d], Carel W. le Roux, PhD[a,*]

KEYWORDS

- Obesity • Bariatric surgery • Weight loss • Metabolic outcomes
- Weight management

KEY POINTS

- Bariatric surgery is an effective treatment modality for obesity and obesity-associated complications.
- Weight loss after bariatric surgery was initially attributed to anatomic restriction or reduced energy absorption, but now it is understood that surgery treats obesity by influencing the subcortical areas of the brain to lower adipose tissue mass.
- There are three major phases of this process: initially the weight loss phase, followed by a phase where weight loss is maintained, and in a subset of patients a phase where weight is regained. These phases are characterized by altered appetitive behavior together with changes in energy expenditure.
- The mechanisms associated with the rearrangement of the gastrointestinal tract include central appetite control, release of gut peptides, change in microbiota and bile acids. However, the exact combination and timing of signals remain largely unknown.

INTRODUCTION

Bariatric surgery is an effective treatment for the disease of obesity and achieves long term weight loss maintenance and health gains.[1–3] Surgery also provided a model offering numerous novel insights on the pathophysiology of obesity.[4] Bariatric surgery procedures do not work primarily by mechanical restriction or causing macronutrient malabsorption, but weight loss is attributed to addressing the pathologic processes causing body weight dysregulation.[5,6] The positive impact on health is predominantly

[a] Diabetes Complications Research Centre, Conway Institute, University College Dublin, Dublin, Ireland; [b] Department of Family Medicine and Polyclinics, King Faisal Specialist Hospital and Research Centre, Riyadh, Saudi Arabia; [c] Altnagelvin Hospital, Derry~Londonderry, UK; [d] School of Medicine, Ulster University, Londonderry, UK
* Corresponding author.
E-mail addresses: khalabduljabbar@kfshrc.edu.sa (K.A.); efstathiosbonanos@windowslive.com (E.B.); a.miras@nhs.net (A.D.M.); carel.leroux@ucd.ie (C.W.R.)

Gastroenterol Clin N Am 52 (2023) 691–705
https://doi.org/10.1016/j.gtc.2023.08.002 gastro.theclinics.com

due to the substantial and sustained weight loss, but there are also weight loss independent mechanisms resulting in health gains.

A growing body of evidence suggests that surgery-induced weight loss is mediated by a complex interplay of factors, including hormonal and bile responses, alterations in gut microbiota, and changes in energy expenditure.[7] A comprehensive understanding of these mechanisms can provide valuable insights into the physiologic basis of weight loss following the surgery, and potentially pave the way for the development of novel therapeutic strategies for obesity and related metabolic disorders.

This review article aims to provide an in-depth analysis of the mechanisms underlying weight loss following bariatric surgery by focusing on mechanistic studies in humans and animal models focusing on Roux-en-Y gastric bypass (RYGB), sleeve gastrectomy (SG) and adjustable gastric banding (AGB). By examining the anatomic and physiologic changes, hormonal and bile responses, gut microbiota alterations, and effects on energy expenditure, this review seeks to offer a holistic perspective on the intricacies of weight loss induced by bariatric surgery.

MECHANISMS RESPONSIBLE FOR WEIGHT LOSS AFTER BARIATRIC SURGERY

Anatomic and Physiologic Changes

Bariatric surgery involves creating a smaller gastric reservoir plus or minus rerouting the small intestine to bypass a portion of the stomach and duodenum.[8,9] This leads to reduced food intake, altered gut hormone and bile secretion, altered gut microbiota, and energy expenditure, all contributing to weight loss. Surgery does not work by creating mechanical restriction or macronutrient malabsorption.[8]

Reduced Food Intake

Reduction in appetitive behavior

An individual's body weight lifetime trajectory is influenced by their genetic make-up, which interacts with non-biological factors (eg, social, psychological) to determine the resulting phenotype.[10] Changes in weight, below or above the individual's usual weight, generate a signal detected by the subcortical areas of the brain, which regulate energy intake and expenditure.[11] When weight loss occurs, a hypoadiposity state signals the depletion of energy stores.[12] An increase in hunger and reduction in satiety is then triggered leading to seeking and consuming food.

Bariatric surgery has proven to be biologically sophisticated and the multiple mechanisms evoked by the surgery may in part be responsible for its effectiveness. During the acute negative energy balance phase, patients after surgery report a decrease in hunger and an increase in satiety while losing weight.[13] The key difference between dieting and bariatric surgery is that after surgery, the body does not recognize the hypoadiposity state as abnormal, but rather it appears as if the goal is to reduce weight by approximately 20% to 30%.[14] Manipulation of the stomach and the small intestine results in favorable changes in humoral and neural signals from the gut to the brain. These signals appear to address the pathologic processes responsible for the disease of obesity.[5] Thus the changes in the humoral and neural milieu maintenance of a new homeostatic state occur at a much lower body adipocyte mass.

Patients' verbal report during the plateau phase of weight loss achieved after bariatric surgery is intriguing. Once the new homeostatic state at a lower body adipocyte mass has been achieved with surgery, patients report an increase in hunger and a decrease in satiety.[15] Although they may have a stable energy balance, patients often have higher energy intake during meals.[16] Despite this, body weight stays the same or increases only marginally. Whilst at this new homeostatic point, the intensity of the internal feelings of hunger and satiety might return to almost pre-operative levels. The surgically altered signaling from the gut acts continuously to treat the disease of obesity. Although total energy intake increases so does energy expenditure, thus allowing defense of the new normal.[15]

Patients losing weight through pharmacotherapy (eg, with glucagon-like peptide 1 (GLP-1) receptor agonists) report very similar changes in their appetite during the acute and chronic phases of their weight loss journey.[17] The only difference is that the effect size of pharmacotherapy is lower than that of surgery. In part this may be because medications change only one or few of the signaling pathways in the appetite centers of the brain.[18]

Weight loss following biliopancreatic diversion or duodenal switch operations emphasizes that the mechanisms underlying the effectiveness of these surgeries are physiologic. These procedures are the most effective operation for weight loss, but rarely performed these days due to the associated nutritional complications. The very long intestinal bypass in this procedure results in macronutrient malabsorption and weight loss, which creates a pathologic hypoadiposity state.[19] The brain appetite centers rapidly detect this and compensate by increasing hunger and food intake. Patients after the biliopancreatic diversion commonly consume more calories compared to before their operation. Despite this, hyperphagia is not enough to compensate for the loss of calories through the gut.[20] The amount of calories loss does not explain the new homeostatic set point which is achieved.[20,21] The calorie malabsorption resulting from the surgery not only limits the impact of hyperphagia but also leads to improvements in the pathologic processes of obesity. In conjunction with the hypo-absorptive state of the small intestine, these factors serve as the dominant mechanisms for weight loss following these procedures.

Neural correlates of reduction in energy intake

The subcortical areas of the brain and for example, the hypothalamus are critical brain areas that control energy intake and expenditure via two sets of antagonistic neurons. Seen in a simplistic way agouti-related peptide (AgRP) neurons promote hunger and pro-opiomelanocortin (POMC) neurons promote satiety.[22] Neuropeptide Y (NPY) is secreted by AgRP neurons and is an orexigenic factor. Hypothalamic gene expression of AgRP, NPY and POMC changes following bariatric surgery but the findings are not consistent and often lack a weight-matched calorie restricted model.[23,24] Expression levels of hypothalamic AgRP in obese female rodents are upregulated when compared to lean controls but go down to levels similar to lean animals following RYGB. During the weight loss phase in the first two postoperative weeks, hypothalamic AgRP and NPY gene expression does not increase compared to mice undergoing sham surgery, suggesting that compensatory hunger signals in the RYGB mice are not activated.[25] In contrast, when the same amount of weight loss was achieved by caloric restriction in a different group of mice, increased expression of AgRP and NPY is observed. POMC expression is not altered to a similar degree as AgRP, indicating that RYGB suppresses the adaptive appetitive response triggered by weight loss.[26–28] Similarly, SG does not change NPY and AgRP gene expression in obese rats during the weight maintenance phase, 4 weeks after surgery.[29] The hypothalamic expression of NPY is significantly lower and the expression of POMC was significantly higher after SG compared to RYGB.[30]

The brainstem is another key player in how bariatric surgery suppresses appetitive behavior. The strong orexigenic drive stemming from arcuate AgRP/NPY neurons may partially result from the inhibition of an equally strong feeding anorexia circuit organized around the lateral parabrachial nucleus (lPBN) and brainstem.[31,32] Measurement of meal-induced neuronal activation by means of c-Fos in obese mice showed that brainstem anorexia circuit may have a potential role in adaptive neural and behavioral changes involved in the strong early suppression of energy intake after RYGB.[33]

These findings from animal models support the observations from humans in that the direction of change in expression of neuropeptides in the hypothalamus and brainstem after RYGB and SG is opposite to caloric restriction through dieting and favor the maintenance of a new homeostatic and lower body weight.[34] Thus the appetite changes may not be responsible for the weight loss, but rather the appetite changes are the response once the pathologic processes of obesity have been addressed and the subcortical areas of the brain are guiding the body to achieve a new homeostasis at a lower body weight. This may also explain why patients report their hunger returning once they achieve the new homeostasis, because the surgery does not influence appetite directly but rather appetite changes are consequences of surgery treating the disease of obesity.

Neural signaling

The mechanism of action of AGB is thought to be predominantly through vagal signaling. Injection of fluid through the subcutaneous port increases the extra-luminal pressure on vagal afferents, sending a signal to the brainstem, even in the fasting state.[35] This mechanism is further exaggerated through the increase in fundal intra-luminal pressure exerted by the consumption of food, leading to early satiety during a meal. These enhanced signals appear to treat the pathologic processes of obesity, leading to weight loss in patients until they reach a new homeostatic body weight. Adding too much fluid into the AGB for patients in cases where the procedure has not effectively treated the pathologic processes of obesity, leads to mechanical restriction and vomiting. This is a preventable complication that should be avoided, and instead an early decision should be made to remove the AGB in patients who do not respond. More patients do not respond to the AGB compared to RYGB/SG.[36,37] This may be because the AGB activates fewer signaling systems to the brain, as opposed to the plethora of signals after RYGB/SG. A study in rats suggested that signals carried by vagal afferents from the mid and lower small intestine contribute to the early RYGB-induced body weight loss and reduction of food intake.[38] Disruption of vagal afferent and/or efferent takes place during RYGB and SG surgery; whether this is sufficient to treat obesity. Some studies suggested that vagal sparing surgical technique affects body weight loss in rodents, and therefore the vagal nerve should be preserved during the RYGB.[39,40] However, there are limited data on the role of vagus nerve dissection in RYGB and SG with regards to body weight in humans.[41]

Food selection

Initially it was thought that after RYGB and SG surgery, but not AGB, some patients changed their food selection to less energy-dense options.[42,43] However, the majority of research in this area used indirect measures of behavior (eg, questionnaires, food diaries and verbal reports) at recall sessions. These methods have large variations in response and substantial heterogeneity in findings.[44] This is particularly noticeable in the longer-term measurements of eating behavior, 5 to 10 years after surgery when any early changes in macronutrient selection tend to dissipate.

Only a small number of studies have used direct measurements of eating behavior, that is, observing the participant's choices during an ad libitum meal or an eating behavior task. The highest quality studies using direct measures of behavior suggest that patients eat the same food and the same number of meals 1 year after surgery but they eat smaller portions.[45] There was an association between weight loss and selection of food with a lower percentage of fat and low-glycemic index foods, and a higher percentage of protein as a proportion of total daily caloric intake.[46]

The reduction in the rewarding properties of food is one of the mechanisms that underpins the changes in food selection. This mechanism has been investigated using functional neuroimaging. Functional Magnetic resonance imaging (MRI) and Positron Emission Tomography (PET) studies suggest both the direction of change and the areas of the brain reward system that correlate with changes in observed or reported eating behavior. Notwithstanding discrepancies between studies, there is some agreement that there is a reduction in the activation of brain areas that respond to the involved cues with rewarding properties to food cues after RYGB and SG.[47,48] This is consistent with the reduced appetitive behavior often seen within the weight loss phase during the first year after surgery. The effect size of this reduction is more pronounced after RYGB compared to SG.[49] Gut hormones are mediators that are associated with this observation, as the blockage of the gut hormones partly reverses the reduction in the activation of these brain regions.[50] This is in line with animal and human data demonstrating that gut hormones such as glucagon-like peptide-1 (GLP-1) and peptide YY (PYY) do not just reduce hunger and increase fullness, but reduce the rewarding properties of food through their direct action on their receptors in brain reward areas.[51] However, the result of neuroimaging should always be interpreted within the context of whether they are performed during the weight loss phase or the phase when the new homeostatic weight is achieved.

The valid measurement of the consummatory reward value of taste is challenging in humans as it relies entirely on the use of indirect measures such as visual analogue scales (VAS). Studies using VAS after RYGB surgery have shown discrepant results.[52,53] There is more consistency in the rodent literature, in which orofacial responses, a good marker of consummatory responses, increase for low concentrations of glucose and decrease for high concentrations of glucose after RYGB.[54,55] The third domain of taste function is termed digestive preparation and salivation is a marker of this reflex response to tastants. Rates of salivation correlate with the rewarding aspects of the tastant and people with obesity demonstrate higher salivation rates to normal-weight controls.[56] Attempts have been made to measure salivation rates after obesity surgery but with mixed results.[57]

Neural signaling also contributes to changes in the rewarding value of fat and sugar after surgery. Obese rats after RYGB produce less of the fat-satiety molecule oleoylethanolamide in the small intestine, and this effect is associated with vagus nerve-driven increases in dorsal striatal dopamine release.[58] When local oleoylethanolamide, vagal, and dorsal striatal dopamine-1 receptor signaling are inhibited, the beneficial effects of RYGB on fat intake and preferences are reversed.

The available data indicate that alterations in food selection occur in a proportion of individuals after RYGB and SG, but not AGB. In the case of RYGB and SG, this mechanism could complement the decrease in hunger and enhanced satiety, resulting in further weight loss. It remains unclear whether this mechanism is sustained over time or diminishes following intestinal adaptation. The impact of learning to avoid foods causing undesirable post-ingestion effects is probably more significant in determining food preferences after surgery than taste function.

Hormonal Responses

Bariatric surgery causes changes in the plasma levels of several gut hormones, which play crucial roles in treating the disease of obesity and in the process changes appetite regulation, glucose homeostasis, and energy expenditure (**Fig. 1**).

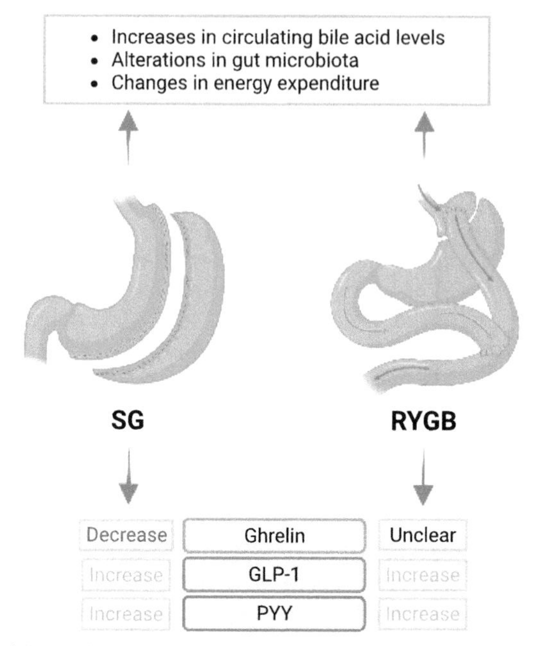

Fig. 1. Changes in bile acids and gut hormones after the common bariatric procedures; SG: sleeve gastrectomy, RYGB: Roux-en-Y gastric bypass, GLP-1: Glucagon-Like Peptide-1, PYY: Peptide YY. (Created with BioRender.com.)

Ghrelin

Ghrelin, is also known as a "hunger hormone," which is predominantly produced by the stomach and binds receptors in the subcortical areas of the brain to stimulate appetitive behavior. Following bariatric surgery, especially SG, the production of ghrelin is significantly reduced due to the exclusion of a large portion of the stomach from the gastrointestinal tract. This reduction in ghrelin levels contributes to decreased hunger.[59,60] The data after RYGB is less clear with studies suggesting increases, decreases, or no change.[61–64]

Satiety gut hormones such as glucagon-like peptide-1 and peptide YY

Following surgery, levels of GLP-1 and PYY increase, leading to increased satiety and reduced food intake.[13] GLP-1 also enhances insulin secretion and sensitivity, improving glucose homeostasis. GLP-1 is an incretin hormone released by the L-cells of the distal small intestine and colon in response to nutrient intake. GLP-1 stimulates insulin secretion from pancreatic beta-cells in a glucose-dependent manner, leading to improved glucose homeostasis. Moreover, GLP-1 increases insulin sensitivity in peripheral tissues, further enhancing glucose utilization.[60,65]

PYY is another gut hormone secreted by the L-cells of the distal small intestine and colon in response to nutrient intake. PYY acts on the subcortical areas of the brain including the hypothalamus, to reduce appetitive behavior and food intake by inhibiting the release of neuropeptide Y (NPY), a potent appetite stimulant. The increased secretion of PYY following surgery contributes to the overall reduction in appetitive behavior and caloric intake.[60,65]

Bile acids

Bariatric surgery increases circulating bile acid levels, which are involved in lipid and glucose metabolism regulation. Bile acids can also stimulate the production of GLP-1 and other hormones, further contributing to weight loss.[66]

Bile acids activate various nuclear and cell surface receptors, such as the farnesoid X receptor (FXR) and the G-protein-coupled bile acid receptor (TGR5). These receptors regulate the expression of genes involved in lipid and glucose metabolism, as well as the secretion of gut hormones, including GLP-1.[67] The increased plasma bile acid levels following bariatric surgery may contribute to improved metabolic regulation and weight loss.

Gut Microbiota Alterations

Bariatric surgery leads to significant changes in gut microbiota composition. These changes include an increase in Bacteroidetes and a decrease in Firmicutes, which are associated with increased energy expenditure and reduced energy harvest from the diet.

Gut microbiota composition and energy harvest

The gut microbiota plays a role in energy harvest and metabolism, with specific bacterial phyla having distinct metabolic profiles.[68] The increased abundance of Bacteroidetes and reduced abundance of Firmicutes observed following surgery have been associated with decreased energy harvest from the diet and increased energy expenditure.[69,70] It is likely that microbiota play a causative role after RYGB, because when the gut microbiota from patients who had RYGB were transplanted to germ free mice, the mice gained less weight compared to the control group.[71]

Short-chain fatty acids

Gut bacteria, particularly those belonging to the phylum Bacteroidetes, ferment dietary fiber and produce short-chain fatty acids (SCFAs) such as acetate, propionate, and butyrate. SCFAs can modulate energy metabolism by acting as signaling molecules and influencing the release of gut hormones, such as GLP-1 and PYY.[72] The shift in gut microbiota composition following surgery may contribute to weight loss through alterations in SCFA production and associated metabolic effects.[73,74]

Effects on Energy Expenditure

Measuring energy expenditure is challenging. Changes in energy expenditure should also be interpreted in the context of total body weight and fat-free mass, both of which are major determinants of total energy expenditure. The components of energy expenditure include basal metabolic rate, non-exercise activity thermogenesis, activity thermogenesis, and diet-associated thermogenesis. All of these may change in different directions depending on a set of signals from a specific stimulus, such as obesity surgery.

Relatively enhanced energy expenditure after bariatric surgery may be a result of the new homeostatic body weight that is achieved. Resting energy expenditure in humans following RYGB using indirect calorimetry show either a decrease within the first postoperative year,[75,76] stability[77] or even slightly increase in the longer term.[78] These changes are reported to be highly dependent on organ-tissue body composition as patients with RYGB maintain a larger high-metabolic rate organ mass than non-operated controls.[77] Moreover, acute weight loss following bariatric surgery was found to affect the accuracy of energy expenditure predictive equations.[79]

A small number of studies used 24-h indirect calorimetry, a method that is optimal for measuring substrate oxidation because each subject can freely move, consume meals, and engage in physical activity. During the rapid weight loss phase, 8 weeks post-treatment, 24-h energy expenditure was significantly decreased from baseline after RYGB, SG, AGB and very low-calorie diet, following adjustment for decreases in fat-free mass and fat mass. However, this effect persisted for up to 1 year after

RYGB and SG (RYGB, −124 ± 42; VSG, −155 ± 118 kcal/d).[80] Another study reported no changes in 24-h or diet-induced energy expenditure, during the rapid weight loss phase, 11 weeks after RYGB, although this was not corrected for total tissue mass.[81] Patients who underwent biliopancreatic diversion (consisting of a horizontal gastrectomy with a distal Roux-en-Y reconstruction resulting in an alimentary limb of 250 cm and a common channel of 50–100 cm) demonstrated increased meal associated related-thermogenesis (11.0% at baseline to 19.9% of caloric intake) and physical activity related-thermogenesis (8344.3 at baseline to 9701.4 kcal/24 hr) during the weight loss phase at 6-month postoperatively, when compared to an unoperated control group.[82] Meal associated energy expenditure in patients during the phase when weight stabilized, 20 months after RYGB, was increased, which resulted in an increased contribution to total energy expenditure over 24 hours from an average of 12.9 cal/min/kg to 14.7 cal/min/kg, when corrected for total tissue mass, including total adipose tissue, lean body mass, bone mineral density and bone mineral content.[83]

Nine years after RYGB, during the phase of weight maintenance, patients had greater meal associated energy expenditure and total 24-h energy expenditure at an average of 16.9 cal/min/kg when compared to Vertical Banded Gastroplasty patients, a procedure similar to AGB, at 14.9 cal/min/kg.[84] One mechanism which may contribute to increased energy expenditure during a meal in humans may be the enhanced glucose utilization by the hypertrophied small intestine.[85] However, absolute energy expenditure is reduced after surgery in humans and the increase in energy expenditure expressed per total body mass may be at least in part explained by the change in body composition (ie, increased lean-to-fat mass ratio).

Contrary to observations in humans, the majority of studies in rodent models of RYGB report an increase in total energy expenditure when compared with ad libitum-fed shams and weight-matched shams. This has been measured at different postoperative time points using indirect calorimetry or validated mathematical formulae.[86–88] SG appears to induce little change in total energy expenditure.[29,87,88] However, indirect calorimetry produces an absolute error as high as 38% when compared with standard direct calorimetry.[89] Using a combination of sensitive direct and indirect calorimetry to overcome this limitation and demonstrated an increase in resting energy expenditure after RYGB, but not SG in rodents.[90]

Brown adipose tissue (BAT) is a major organ regulating energy metabolism by thermogenesis and triglyceride clearance and plays a role in energy expenditure changes after obesity surgery.[91,92] A decrease in triglyceride content, together with the increased proportion of brown adipose tissue in the supraclavicular fat depot was found in women 6 months after RYGB and SG.[93] The role of BAT in energy expenditure following bariatric surgery has mainly been studied in rodents. Expression of key BAT thermoregulatory genes, such as uncoupling protein-1 (UCP-1), remain unchanged following RYGB but are reduced in caloric-restricted weight-matched animals,[94] and that the bypassed duodenum has a key role in the observed postoperative metabolic profile.[95] The volume and metabolic activity of BAT, as recorded by micro-positron emission tomography/computed tomography, increased following RYGB, but not after AGB and SG.[96] A mechanism underlying the metabolic activity of BAT is the increase in growth hormone/insulin-like growth factor-1, which regulates adipocyte differentiation.[96] Unlike SG, RYGB causes an increase in total resting metabolic rate, as well as a specific increase in splanchnic sympathetic nerve activity and "browning" of visceral mesenteric fat via endocannabinoid signaling within the small intestine.[90] Although in vivo studies are vital to unravel the mechanisms of energy expenditure difference after obesity surgery, it is important to note the species difference between mice and rats, as well as strain differences in a single species. There are also differences between rodent and human BAT, in terms of depot locations, beige and brown adipose tissue amount and thermogenic capacity.[97] Despite this, UCP1 content and function are similar between human and mouse BAT.[98]

Overall, it appears unlikely that postoperative weight loss is driven by enhanced energy expenditure after RYGB and SG, but the changes in energy expenditure during the phase when weight loss stabilizes suggest that the subcortical areas of the brain may have reached a new homeostasis and hence there is an attenuation of the reduction in energy expenditure which can be associated with weight loss resulting in a non-homeostatic hypoadiposity state. The differences in energy expenditure discussed above could be due to differences in diet, patient body composition and energy expenditure measurement. Taken together the contribution of energy expenditure to weight loss after RYGB and SG is less than the effect of food intake in humans, albeit in rodents energy expenditure may be more important.

Weight Regain

Although bariatric surgery results in substantial and sustained weight loss for many patients, a subset of individuals may experience weight regain in the long term. Observational studies have reported that 10% to 20% of patients regain a significant amount of weight within 5 to 10 years after surgery.[99] Previously factors such as dietary habits, physical activity levels, and psychological factors were considered as contributors, but now weight regain may be considered as a response in a subset of patients, where bariatric surgery is no longer able to control the disease of obesity. Thus in these patients, weight regain represents escape of the disease in a similar way cancer may escape surgical control. Identifying patients at risk of weight regain and providing appropriate interventions remain challenging as currently no predictors exist.

SUMMARY

The anatomic manipulations during the most frequently used bariatric procedures treat the disease of obesity through a complex interplay of factors, including hormonal and bile responses, alterations in gut microbiota, and changes in energy expenditure. A new homeostatic body weight can only be achieved by an initial reduction in appetite. When the new homeostatic weight is achieved then appetite and energy expenditure return but remain in balance to maintain the new adipose tissue mass. Altered signaling from the gut to the brain, the major organ contributing to the disease of obesity, facilitates the treatment of the disease of obesity. Unraveling of the elusive physiology of the gut after bariatric surgery will not only help optimize surgical procedures, develop nonsurgical therapies, address weight regain after surgery, but will also aid the understanding of the pathophysiology of the disease of obesity itself.

CLINIC CARE POINTS

- The weight loss after bariatric surgery is biologically determined and at the moment it is not possible to predict weight loss on the patient's motivation or demographics.
- If a patient does not have a good response to bariatric surgery within the first year then it is unlikely because the surgical procedure was not good or because of something the patient did but it is more likely due to the biology of the disease of obesity.
- Long term weight maintenance remain the most common outcome after surgery, but in those who regain weight, additional nutritional therapies and or pharmacotherapy should be considered as soon as possible to maintain as much of the weight lost after surgery.

REFERENCES

1. Adams TD, Davidson LE, Litwin SE, et al. Weight and Metabolic Outcomes 12 Years after Gastric Bypass. N Engl J Med 2017;377(12):1143–55.
2. Courcoulas AP, Yanovski SZ, Bonds D, et al. Long-term outcomes of bariatric surgery: a National Institutes of Health symposium. JAMA Surg 2014;149(12): 1323–9.
3. Arterburn DE, Olsen MK, Smith VA, et al. Association between bariatric surgery and long-term survival. JAMA 2015;313(1):62–70.
4. Ciobârcă D, Cătoi AF, Copăescu C, et al. Bariatric Surgery in Obesity: Effects on Gut Microbiota and Micronutrient Status. Nutrients 2020;12(1):235.
5. le Roux CW, Bueter M. The physiology of altered eating behaviour after Roux-en-Y gastric bypass. Exp Physiol 2014;99(9):1128–32.
6. Batterham RL, Cummings DE. Mechanisms of Diabetes Improvement Following Bariatric/Metabolic Surgery. Diabetes Care 2016;39(6):893–901.
7. Puzziferri N, Roshek TB 3rd, Mayo HG, et al. Long-term follow-up after bariatric surgery: a systematic review. JAMA 2014;312(9):934–42.
8. Buchwald H, Avidor Y, Braunwald E, et al. Bariatric surgery: a systematic review and meta-analysis. JAMA 2004;292(14):1724–37.
9. Brethauer SA, Hammel JP, Schauer PR. Systematic review of sleeve gastrectomy as staging and primary bariatric procedure. Surg Obes Relat Dis 2009;5(4): 469–75.
10. Farias MM, Cuevas AM, Rodriguez F. Set-point theory and obesity. Metab Syndr Relat Disord 2011;9(2):85–9.
11. Woods SC, D'Alessio DA. Central control of body weight and appetite. J Clin Endocrinol Metab 2008;93(11 Suppl 1):S37–50.
12. Rosenbaum M, Leibel RL. Adaptive thermogenesis in humans. Int J Obes 2010; 34(Suppl 1):S47–55.
13. le Roux CW, Aylwin SJ, Batterham RL, et al. Gut hormone profiles following bariatric surgery favor an anorectic state, facilitate weight loss, and improve metabolic parameters. Ann Surg 2006;243(1):108–14.
14. Laurenius A, Larsson I, Melanson KJ, et al. Decreased energy density and changes in food selection following Roux-en-Y gastric bypass. Eur J Clin Nutr 2013;67(2):168–73.
15. Sumithran P, Prendergast LA, Delbridge E, et al. Long-term persistence of hormonal adaptations to weight loss. N Engl J Med 2011;365(17):1597–604.
16. Laurenius A, Larsson I, Bueter M, et al. Changes in eating behaviour and meal pattern following Roux-en-Y gastric bypass. Int J Obes 2012;36(3):348–55.
17. Blundell J, Finlayson G, Axelsen M, et al. Effects of once-weekly semaglutide on appetite, energy intake, control of eating, food preference and body weight in subjects with obesity. Diabetes Obes Metab 2017;19(9):1242–51.
18. Wen X, Zhang B, Wu B, et al. Signaling pathways in obesity: mechanisms and therapeutic interventions. Signal Transduct Target Ther 2022;7(1):298.
19. Anderson B, Gill RS, de Gara CJ, et al. Biliopancreatic diversion: the effectiveness of duodenal switch and its limitations. Gastroenterol Res Pract 2013;2013: 974762.
20. Adami GF, Gandolfo P, Dapueto R, et al. Eating behavior following biliopancreatic diversion for obesity: study with a three-factor eating questionnaire. Int J Eat Disord 1993;14(1):81–6.
21. Pilkington TR, Gazet JC, Ang L, et al. Explanations for weight loss after ileojejunal bypass in gross obesity. Br Med J 1976;1(6024):1504–5.

22. Schwartz MW, Woods SC, Porte D Jr, et al. Central nervous system control of food intake. Nature 2000;404(6778):661–71.
23. Cavin JB, Voitellier E, Cluzeaud F, et al. Malabsorption and intestinal adaptation after one anastomosis gastric bypass compared with Roux-en-Y gastric bypass in rats. Am J Physiol Gastrointest Liver Physiol 2016;311(3):G492–500.
24. Barkholt P, Pedersen PJ, Hay-Schmidt A, et al. Alterations in hypothalamic gene expression following Roux-en-Y gastric bypass. Mol Metab 2016;5(4):296–304.
25. Herrick MK, Favela KM, Simerly RB, et al. Attenuation of diet-induced hypothalamic inflammation following bariatric surgery in female mice. Mol Med 2018; 24(1):56.
26. Patkar PP, Hao Z, Mumphrey MB, et al. Unlike calorie restriction, Roux-en-Y gastric bypass surgery does not increase hypothalamic AgRP and NPY in mice on a high-fat diet. Int J Obes 2019;43(11):2143–50.
27. Nadreau E, Baraboi ED, Samson P, et al. Effects of the biliopancreatic diversion on energy balance in the rat. Int J Obes 2006;30(3):419–29.
28. Turnbaugh PJ, Ley RE, Mahowald MA, et al. An obesity-associated gut microbiome with increased capacity for energy harvest. Nature 2006;444(7122): 1027–31.
29. Stefater MA, Pérez-Tilve D, Chambers AP, et al. Sleeve gastrectomy induces loss of weight and fat mass in obese rats, but does not affect leptin sensitivity. Gastroenterology 2010;138(7):2426–36, 2436.e1-3.
30. Kawasaki T, Ohta M, Kawano Y, et al. Effects of sleeve gastrectomy and gastric banding on the hypothalamic feeding center in an obese rat model. Surg Today 2015;45(12):1560–6.
31. Atasoy D, Betley JN, Su HH, et al. Deconstruction of a neural circuit for hunger. Nature 2012;488(7410):172–7.
32. Sternson SM. Hypothalamic survival circuits: blueprints for purposive behaviors. Neuron 2013;77(5):810–24.
33. Mumphrey MB, Hao Z, Townsend RL, et al. Eating in mice with gastric bypass surgery causes exaggerated activation of brainstem anorexia circuit. Int J Obes 2016;40(6):921–8.
34. Martinou E, Stefanova I, Iosif E, et al. Neurohormonal Changes in the Gut-Brain Axis and Underlying Neuroendocrine Mechanisms following Bariatric Surgery. Int J Mol Sci 2022;23(6).
35. Stefanidis A, Forrest N, Brown WA, et al. An investigation of the neural mechanisms underlying the efficacy of the adjustable gastric band. Surg Obes Relat Dis 2016;12(4):828–38.
36. Arterburn D, Powers JD, Toh S, et al. Comparative effectiveness of laparoscopic adjustable gastric banding vs laparoscopic gastric bypass. JAMA Surg 2014; 149(12):1279–87.
37. Chang SH, Stoll CR, Song J, et al. The effectiveness and risks of bariatric surgery: an updated systematic review and meta-analysis, 2003-2012. JAMA Surg 2014; 149(3):275–87.
38. Hao Z, Townsend RL, Mumphrey MB, et al. Vagal innervation of intestine contributes to weight loss After Roux-en-Y gastric bypass surgery in rats. Obes Surg 2014;24(12):2145–51.
39. Bueter M, Löwenstein C, Ashrafian H, et al. Vagal sparing surgical technique but not stoma size affects body weight loss in rodent model of gastric bypass. Obes Surg 2010;20(5):616–22.

40. Ballsmider LA, Vaughn AC, David M, et al. Sleeve gastrectomy and Roux-en-Y gastric bypass alter the gut-brain communication. Neural Plast 2015;2015: 601985.
41. Perathoner A, Weiss H, Santner W, et al. Vagal nerve dissection during pouch formation in laparoscopic Roux-Y-gastric bypass for technical simplification: does it matter? Obes Surg 2009;19(4):412–7.
42. Halmi KA, Mason E, Falk JR, et al. Appetitive behavior after gastric bypass for obesity. Int J Obes 1981;5(5):457–64.
43. Gero D, Steinert RE, le Roux CW, et al. Do Food Preferences Change After Bariatric Surgery? Curr Atheroscler Rep 2017;19(9):38.
44. Mathes CM, Spector AC. Food selection and taste changes in humans after Roux-en-Y gastric bypass surgery: a direct-measures approach. Physiol Behav 2012;107(4):476–83.
45. Livingstone MBE, Redpath T, Naseer F, et al. Food Intake Following Gastric Bypass Surgery: Patients Eat Less but Do Not Eat Differently. J Nutr 2022; 152(11):2319–32.
46. Nielsen MS, Christensen BJ, Ritz C, et al. Roux-En-Y Gastric Bypass and Sleeve Gastrectomy Does Not Affect Food Preferences When Assessed by an Ad libitum Buffet Meal. Obes Surg 2017;27(10):2599–605.
47. Scholtz S, Miras AD, Chhina N, et al. Obese patients after gastric bypass surgery have lower brain-hedonic responses to food than after gastric banding. Gut 2014; 63(6):891–902.
48. Baboumian S, Pantazatos SP, Kothari S, et al. Functional Magnetic Resonance Imaging (fMRI) of Neural Responses to Visual and Auditory Food Stimuli Pre and Post Roux-en-Y Gastric Bypass (RYGB) and Sleeve Gastrectomy (SG). Neuroscience 2019;409:290–8.
49. Smith KR, Papantoni A, Veldhuizen MG, et al. Taste-related reward is associated with weight loss following bariatric surgery. J Clin Invest 2020;130(8):4370–81.
50. Goldstone AP, Miras AD, Scholtz S, et al. Link Between Increased Satiety Gut Hormones and Reduced Food Reward After Gastric Bypass Surgery for Obesity. J Clin Endocrinol Metab 2016;101(2):599–609.
51. De Silva A, Salem V, Long CJ, et al. The gut hormones PYY 3-36 and GLP-1 7-36 amide reduce food intake and modulate brain activity in appetite centers in humans. Cell Metab 2011;14(5):700–6.
52. Bueter M, Miras AD, Chichger H, et al. Alterations of sucrose preference after Roux-en-Y gastric bypass. Physiol Behav 2011;104(5):709–21.
53. Pepino MY, Bradley D, Eagon JC, et al. Changes in taste perception and eating behavior after bariatric surgery-induced weight loss in women. Obesity 2014; 22(5):E13–20.
54. Shin AC, Zheng H, Pistell PJ, et al. Roux-en-Y gastric bypass surgery changes food reward in rats. Int J Obes 2011;35(5):642–51.
55. Berthoud HR, Zheng H, Shin AC. Food reward in the obese and after weight loss induced by calorie restriction and bariatric surgery. Ann N Y Acad Sci 2012; 1264(1):36–48.
56. Bond DS, Raynor HA, Vithiananthan S, et al. Differences in salivary habituation to a taste stimulus in bariatric surgery candidates and normal-weight controls. Obes Surg 2009;19(7):873–8.
57. Farias T, Vasconcelos B, SoutoMaior JR, et al. Influence of Bariatric Surgery on Salivary Flow: a Systematic Review and Meta-Analysis. Obes Surg 2019;29(5): 1675–80.

58. Hankir MK, Seyfried F, Hintschich CA, et al. Gastric Bypass Surgery Recruits a Gut PPAR-α-Striatal D1R Pathway to Reduce Fat Appetite in Obese Rats. Cell Metab 2017;25(2):335–44.
59. Meek CL, Lewis HB, Reimann F, et al. The effect of bariatric surgery on gastrointestinal and pancreatic peptide hormones. Peptides 2016;77:28–37.
60. Perakakis N, Kokkinos A, Peradze N, et al. Circulating levels of gastrointestinal hormones in response to the most common types of bariatric surgery and predictive value for weight loss over one year: Evidence from two independent trials. Metabolism 2019;101:153997.
61. Garcia-Fuentes E, Garrido-Sanchez L, Garcia-Almeida JM, et al. Different effect of laparoscopic Roux-en-Y gastric bypass and open biliopancreatic diversion of Scopinaro on serum PYY and ghrelin levels. Obes Surg 2008;18(11):1424–9.
62. Pérez-Romero N, Serra A, Granada ML, et al. Effects of two variants of Roux-en-Y Gastric bypass on metabolism behaviour: focus on plasma ghrelin concentrations over a 2-year follow-up. Obes Surg 2010;20(5):600–9.
63. Cummings DE, Weigle DS, Frayo RS, et al. Plasma ghrelin levels after diet-induced weight loss or gastric bypass surgery. N Engl J Med 2002;346(21):1623–30.
64. Korner J, Inabnet W, Febres G, et al. Prospective study of gut hormone and metabolic changes after adjustable gastric banding and Roux-en-Y gastric bypass. Int J Obes 2009;33(7):786–95.
65. Papamargaritis D, le Roux CW. Do Gut Hormones Contribute to Weight Loss and Glycaemic Outcomes after Bariatric Surgery? Nutrients 2021;13(3).
66. Risstad H, Kristinsson JA, Fagerland MW, et al. Bile acid profiles over 5 years after gastric bypass and duodenal switch: results from a randomized clinical trial. Surg Obes Relat Dis 2017;13(9):1544–53.
67. Albaugh VL, Banan B, Antoun J, et al. Role of Bile Acids and GLP-1 in Mediating the Metabolic Improvements of Bariatric Surgery. Gastroenterology 2019;156(4):1041–51.e1044.
68. Rowland I, Gibson G, Heinken A, et al. Gut microbiota functions: metabolism of nutrients and other food components. Eur J Nutr 2018;57(1):1–24.
69. Palmisano S, Campisciano G, Silvestri M, et al. Changes in Gut Microbiota Composition after Bariatric Surgery: a New Balance to Decode. J Gastrointest Surg 2020;24(8):1736–46.
70. Campisciano G, Palmisano S, Cason C, et al. Gut microbiota characterisation in obese patients before and after bariatric surgery. Benef Microbes 2018;9(3):367–73.
71. Tremaroli V, Karlsson F, Werling M, et al. Roux-en-Y Gastric Bypass and Vertical Banded Gastroplasty Induce Long-Term Changes on the Human Gut Microbiome Contributing to Fat Mass Regulation. Cell Metab 2015;22(2):228–38.
72. Kaji I, Karaki S, Kuwahara A. Short-chain fatty acid receptor and its contribution to glucagon-like peptide-1 release. Digestion 2014;89(1):31–6.
73. Martínez-Sánchez MA, Balaguer-Román A, Fernández-Ruiz VE, et al. Plasma short-chain fatty acid changes after bariatric surgery in patients with severe obesity. Surg Obes Relat Dis 2023;19(7):727–34.
74. Seganfredo FB, Blume CA, Moehlecke M, et al. Weight-loss interventions and gut microbiota changes in overweight and obese patients: a systematic review. Obes Rev 2017;18(8):832–51.
75. Lamarca F, Melendez-Araújo MS, Porto de Toledo I, et al. Relative Energy Expenditure Decreases during the First Year after Bariatric Surgery: A Systematic Review and Meta-Analysis. Obes Surg 2019;29(8):2648–59.

76. Wolfe BM, Schoeller DA, McCrady-Spitzer SK, et al. Resting Metabolic Rate, Total Daily Energy Expenditure, and Metabolic Adaptation 6 Months and 24 Months After Bariatric Surgery. Obesity 2018;26(5):862–8.
77. Heshka S, Lemos T, Astbury NM, et al. Resting Energy Expenditure and Organ-Tissue Body Composition 5 Years After Bariatric Surgery. Obes Surg 2020;30(2):587–94.
78. Wilms B, Ernst B, Thurnheer M, et al. Resting energy expenditure after Roux-en Y gastric bypass surgery. Surg Obes Relat Dis 2018;14(2):191–9.
79. Ravelli MN, Schoeller DA, Crisp AH, et al. Accuracy of total energy expenditure predictive equations after a massive weight loss induced by bariatric surgery. Clin Nutr ESPEN 2018;26:57–65.
80. Tam CS, Redman LM, Greenway F, et al. Energy Metabolic Adaptation and Cardiometabolic Improvements One Year After Gastric Bypass, Sleeve Gastrectomy, and Gastric Band. J Clin Endocrinol Metab 2016;101(10):3755–64.
81. Schmidt JB, Pedersen SD, Gregersen NT, et al. Effects of RYGB on energy expenditure, appetite and glycaemic control: a randomized controlled clinical trial. Int J Obes 2016;40(2):281–90.
82. Iesari S, le Roux CW, De Gaetano A, et al. Twenty-four hour energy expenditure and skeletal muscle gene expression changes after bariatric surgery. J Clin Endocrinol Metab 2013;98(2):E321–7.
83. Werling M, Fändriks L, Olbers T, et al. Roux-en-Y Gastric Bypass Surgery Increases Respiratory Quotient and Energy Expenditure during Food Intake. PLoS One 2015;10(6):e0129784.
84. Werling M, Olbers T, Fändriks L, et al. Increased postprandial energy expenditure may explain superior long term weight loss after Roux-en-Y gastric bypass compared to vertical banded gastroplasty. PLoS One 2013;8(4):e60280.
85. Saeidi N, Meoli L, Nestoridi E, et al. Reprogramming of intestinal glucose metabolism and glycemic control in rats after gastric bypass. Science 2013;341(6144):406–10.
86. Bueter M, Löwenstein C, Olbers T, et al. Gastric bypass increases energy expenditure in rats. Gastroenterology 2010;138(5):1845–53.
87. Hao Z, Townsend RL, Mumphrey MB, et al. RYGB Produces more Sustained Body Weight Loss and Improvement of Glycemic Control Compared with VSG in the Diet-Induced Obese Mouse Model. Obes Surg 2017;27(9):2424–33.
88. Stylopoulos N, Hoppin AG, Kaplan LM. Roux-en-Y gastric bypass enhances energy expenditure and extends lifespan in diet-induced obese rats. Obesity 2009;17(10):1839–47.
89. Walsberg GE, Hoffman TC. Direct calorimetry reveals large errors in respirometric estimates of energy expenditure. J Exp Biol 2005;208(Pt 6):1035–43.
90. Ye Y, Abu El Haija M, Morgan DA, et al. Endocannabinoid Receptor-1 and Sympathetic Nervous System Mediate the Beneficial Metabolic Effects of Gastric Bypass. Cell Rep 2020;33(4):108270.
91. Cypess AM, Lehman S, Williams G, et al. Identification and importance of brown adipose tissue in adult humans. N Engl J Med 2009;360(15):1509–17.
92. Bartelt A, Bruns OT, Reimer R, et al. Brown adipose tissue activity controls triglyceride clearance. Nat Med 2011;17(2):200–5.
93. Dadson P, Hannukainen JC, Din MU, et al. Brown adipose tissue lipid metabolism in morbid obesity: Effect of bariatric surgery-induced weight loss. Diabetes Obes Metab 2018;20(5):1280–8.

94. Hankir MK, Bronisch F, Hintschich C, et al. Differential effects of Roux-en-Y gastric bypass surgery on brown and beige adipose tissue thermogenesis. Metabolism 2015;64(10):1240–9.
95. Baraboi ED, Li W, Labbé SM, et al. Metabolic changes induced by the biliopancreatic diversion in diet-induced obesity in male rats: the contributions of sleeve gastrectomy and duodenal switch. Endocrinology 2015;156(4):1316–29.
96. Chen Y, Yang J, Nie X, et al. Effects of Bariatric Surgery on Change of Brown Adipocyte Tissue and Energy Metabolism in Obese Mice. Obes Surg 2018;28(3):820–30.
97. Vosselman MJ, van Marken Lichtenbelt WD, Schrauwen P. Energy dissipation in brown adipose tissue: from mice to men. Mol Cell Endocrinol 2013;379(1–2):43–50.
98. Porter C, Herndon DN, Chondronikola M, et al. Human and Mouse Brown Adipose Tissue Mitochondria Have Comparable UCP1 Function. Cell Metab 2016;24(2):246–55.
99. Athanasiadis DI, Martin A, Kapsampelis P, et al. Factors associated with weight regain post-bariatric surgery: a systematic review. Surg Endosc 2021;35(8):4069–84.

Surgical Management of Bariatric Complications and Weight Regain

Kelvin Higa, MD

KEYWORDS

- Weight loss • Weight regain • Sleeve gastrectomy • Marginal ulcers
- Revision bariatric surgery

KEY POINTS

- Bariatric/Metabolic procedures are safe and effective; complications are rare but should be managed in the appropriate centers of expertise.
- Surgical treatment for inadequate weight loss and /or weight gain should involve evaluation and optimization of the individual's anatomy.
- Decreasing total alimentary limb length may impart a greater metabolic response, but at the risk of malabsorption.

The history and evolution of bariatric/metabolic surgical procedures allows for only a brief introduction to complications and surgical approaches for improved weight loss. Our specialty lacks standardization of our operations such as gastric pouch size, intestinal bypass lengths, and consensus on which procedure is best for each individual patient. Anatomic construct as well as adherence to lifestyle modifications can affect short- and long-term outcomes. The indications for performing metabolic/bariatric surgery are expanding, and the adoption of new innovative operations has added to the complexity of caring for these patients.

COMPLICATIONS

General considerations: With the advent of minimally invasive techniques, overall morbidity and mortality of bariatric surgery has improved considerably over the last 20 years. Early postoperative complications that may require surgical intervention include thromboembolism, leakage, bleeding, and bowel obstruction. Most of our patients are at least moderate risk for thromboembolism and therefore both mechanical and chemical prophylaxis is recommended.[1] Peculiar to the sleeve gastrectomy (SG), superior mesenteric or portal vein thrombosis occurs with greater frequency than other procedures.[2] The exact pathophysiology is unknown, and therefore, targeting

Fresno, CA, USA
E-mail address: higanoid@gmail.com

Gastroenterol Clin N Am 52 (2023) 707–717
https://doi.org/10.1016/j.gtc.2023.09.003
0889-8553/23/

specific patients for postoperative anticoagulation is not possible beyond the usual risk calculators. Depending on the severity of symptoms and potential for bowel ischemia, surgical thrombectomy or catheter-based thrombolysis may be required.[3]

GI leaks outcome benchmarks of RYGB and SG are less than 1.3 and less than 0.15, respectively, for primary bariatric surgery, and 3.5% for elective secondary bariatric surgery.[4] Early postoperative leaks require emergent attention. Patients can often present with minimal symptoms of pain and the physical examination can be unrevealing. Postoperative noninvasive tests such as computerized tomography (CT) or contrast studies can be misleading. Intra-abdominal drains may or may not be indicative of a leak. At times, the only significant finding that dictates reexploration is sustained, unexplained tachycardia.[5] Exploratory laparoscopy should be considered, both as a diagnostic and therapeutic tool. In the case of early leakage, drainage, intraluminal stenting, and establishment of a mechanism for enteric nutrition should be the objectives. Early recognition and treatment will prevent long-term disability and sepsis.[6]

Leaks after SG are often anatomic and related to inexperience. Any twist, kink or narrowing of the midbody of the sleeve can cause a fistula at the angle of His due to high pressure and an "at risk" staple-line. This serious complication can present early, with peritonitis, or subacutely with a chronic abscess. Early fistulas require operative drainage and attempts at reducing the pressure gradient across the sleeve. This can be done with a covered intraluminal stent that must transverse the pylorus and the esophago-gastric (EG) junction. This may require placing two "nesting" stents if a long stent is not available. This is off label use of the stents but is the most common salvage procedure. A seromyotomy of the stomach or balloon dilation might be able to salvage the sleeve, but often conversion to a low-pressure system is required. If the abscess is more chronic and contained, then septotomy, double J stents with combined balloon dilation of the distal stricture, is preferred over operative drainage.[7]

Subacute leaks/fistulas are best managed endoscopically, not by surgery. An example of this is the typical fistula/abscess at the angle of His after SG. This is usually due to a technical problem with relative stenosis at the incisura of the stomach when creating the sleeve. This relative stricture causes a high-pressure staple-line failure that does not present until weeks after surgery. Correction requires both correction of the stenosis, usually with high-pressure balloon dilation and intraluminal drainage with double pig-tailed catheter or endoscopic septotomy. This approach is a paradigm shift in the management of chronic fistulas but is not universally available due to lack of experience and training.[8] As a last resort, conversion to gastric bypass can be performed but should be done only in centers with a high degree of experience.

Bleeding can be either intraluminal or extraluminal, and re-intervention depends on the stability of the patient. Hemodynamic compromise dictates reexploration even if the actual source of bleeding cannot be determined.

Bowel obstruction after any intestinal bypass procedure should be considered a surgical emergency. After gastric bypass, one-anastomosis gastric bypass, duodenal switch, or any procedure where there is a potential for a closed-loop obstruction, the usual general surgical approach of nasogastric decompression is ineffectual and should be avoided. Immediate operative decompression and resolution of the cause of the obstruction is the standard of care. Bariatric surgical patients presenting to institutions without experience will often lead to delay in care and disastrous consequences. In addition, internal hernias, more frequent after laparoscopic procedures due to lack of adhesions, can often present only with pain and no evidence for bowel obstruction by CT or upper gastro intestinal (UGI). The typical "swirl sign" due to mesenteric volvulus and other findings can be absent in up to 20%

of patients, despite impending bowel infarction.[9] Therefore, any patient after gastric bypass requires an exploration for unexplained abdominal pain to rule out internal hernias or other causes of pain.

Marginal ulceration can occur early or late after bariatric surgery. Typical presentation is that of dyspepsia, pain, nausea, or obstruction due to chronic inflammation. Untreated, they can go on to perforate, cause fistulas or bleed. Marginal ulcers are more frequent in individuals who use tobacco or non-steroidal anti-inflamatory drugs (NSAIDs) and are associated with acid exposure to unprotected mucosa such as the gastrojejunostomy after gastric bypass. Nonsurgical treatment requires elimination of tobacco and NSAIDs if possible, proton-pump inhibitors, and surgery for refractory disease.[10]

Perforated marginal ulcers are best treated by emergent laparoscopic exploration and omental patch and drainage. Enteral feedings are most often not necessary as these heal rather quickly. In the convalescent phase, it is important to optimize nutrition, rule out a gastro-gastric fistula, and document complete healing of the ulcer by endoscopy.[11] Nonhealing chronic or recurrent marginal ulcers require surgical intervention. Revision or reversal of the gastric bypass should be made at the recommendation of the multidisciplinary team with the patient included in the shared decision process.

The reversal of gastric bypass procedures is associated with a relatively high complication rate and can lead to other issues such as delayed gastric emptying due to vagal nerve injury, reflux, and weight regain.[12] Conversion to SG is an option, but similar side-effects, especially reflux, acid, and bile, are common and it is difficult to configure a proper sleeve after bypass in one stage due to ischemia of crossing staple lines; therefore, this type of conversion is best done in two stages or utilization of a “jejunal bridge.”[13]

If it is decided that keeping the gastric bypass is the best option, then the surgical goal should be to eliminate acid exposure to the gastrojejunostomy. This requires near complete resection of the gastric pouch, eliminating gastro-gastric fistula if present. Esophagojejunostomy or “near esophagojejunostomy” is the most definitive procedure to reduce the risk of recurrent marginal ulceration.[14]

Malnutrition, malabsorption, dumping syndrome: Most gastrointestinal complications, especially, postprandial hypoglycemia (late dumping syndrome) can be controlled with patient compliance following typical diet plans.[15] However, procedures involving greater percentages of intestinal bypass are more prone to malabsorption and diarrhea. If indicated, surgical correction is aimed at increasing total alimentary limb length (intestine not bypassed) or complete reversal depending on the patient. Systemic stress such as joint replacement or gastroenteritis can lead to protein–calorie malnutrition in patients otherwise stable after biliopancreatic diversion or duodenal switch. As a result of the significant reduction in total alimentary limb length, enteral nutrition will not reverse this entity. These patients can often be salvaged with a few months of parenteral nutrition, but at times, surgery may be necessary to increase the total alimentary length or complete reversal in extreme cases.[16]

INADEQUATE WEIGHT LOSS AND WEIGHT REGAIN

Suboptimal weight loss after surgery is often mistakenly attributed to patient nonadherence and exemplifies obesity bias that exists among health care professionals. It is not logical that an individual would consciously choose to undergo a major irreversible operation to lose weight and then purposely choose a lifestyle for which they understand undermines that very objective. It is more likely that our understanding of the homeostatic mechanisms that preserve a given fat mass set point is still in its infancy and that we lack the precision to predict outcomes, let alone the best operation for a given patient. Rather than blame the patient for inadequate weight loss and burden them with remedial nutritional counseling, efforts should be directed at augmenting, enhancing, or converting their current anatomy for greater effect. Unfortunately, this is not so easy as to try a new medication and most revision procedures are associated with risks far greater than the original operation. Once again, this underscores the importance of choosing, not the best operation for a given patient at a given point in time, but the best option that can be modified in the future for more weight loss, co-morbidity resolution and other unforeseen environmental or social issues.

The approach to a patient with *suboptimal initial weight loss* requires optimization of the patient's understanding and adherence with basic dietary guidelines and investigation of the existing anatomy. Was the operation within normally agreed on specifications, or a result of inexperience or lack of proper training? A detailed history can help determine if the issue is primarily psychological (stress eating/addictive behavioral) or biological (insatiable appetite, hunger).

If it is determined that suboptimal anatomy is the issue, such as a large gastric pouch, then surgical therapy can include corrective measures, that is, pouch reduction via surgery or endoscopy may improve performance. However, if the existing anatomy cannot be improved on, then the best option would be conversion to a more aggressive procedure. These decisions require a thorough evaluation of the patient's nutritional status and risk/benefit analysis.

Weight regain after an initial good response to surgery is often attributed to a major psychosocial event that causes maladaptive eating habits to reappear, but in reality, the reason(s) for this phenomenon is speculative. Anatomic causes, such as the development of a gastro-gastric fistula after gastric bypass, are rare. In these cases, we look to augment or convert to a more aggressive operation, when appropriate.

ADJUSTABLE GASTRIC BAND

The adjustable gastric band (AGB) remains somewhat of an enigma. It remains a viable option but used infrequently for a variety of reasons.[17] Complications of the band are largely port site-related. Owing to a poor design, flipping of the port, making it inaccessible for adjustment requires a minor procedure. Slippage of the band can lead to reflux, food intolerance, weight regain, or acute prolapse of the proximal stomach sometimes requiring emergent surgery to avoid ischemic necrosis of the fundus of the stomach. Erosion of the band through the gastric wall is rarely a surgical emergency but can present with weight regain with no other symptoms. The treatment of erosion requires the removal of the band. This can be accomplished endoscopically or surgically (**Fig. 1**).[18]

Conversion of the AGB can be performed in one- or two-staged procedures. The most common conversions would be to SG or gastric bypass. In this situation, the gastric bypass seems to be associated with better weight loss and less symptomatic GERD than the sleeve, but one must consider the potential need for an even more aggressive operation such as the duodenal switch in the future.[19]

SLEEVE GASTRECTOMY

SG is the most common bariatric procedure worldwide.[20] It is safe, highly effective and has a short learning curve when compared with bypass procedures. Whereas options for weight gain after gastric bypass are limited or highly complex, the SG can be easily converted to the more effective duodenal switch procedures. Conversion of SG

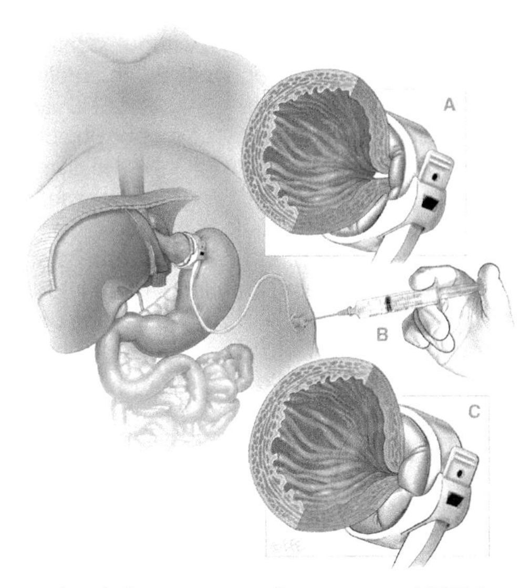

Fig. 1. Adjustable gastric band. (© Dr Levent Efe, courtesy of IFSO.)

to gastric bypass for additional weight loss has been disappointing and likely to due to the similar biochemical effects of each procedure.[21] Re-SG has been reported but with mixed results.[22] Conversion of SG to one-anastomosis gastric bypass may have better performance than Roux-en-Y gastric bypass (RYGB), depending on the magnitude of intestinal bypass (biliopancreatic limb) used (**Fig. 2**).

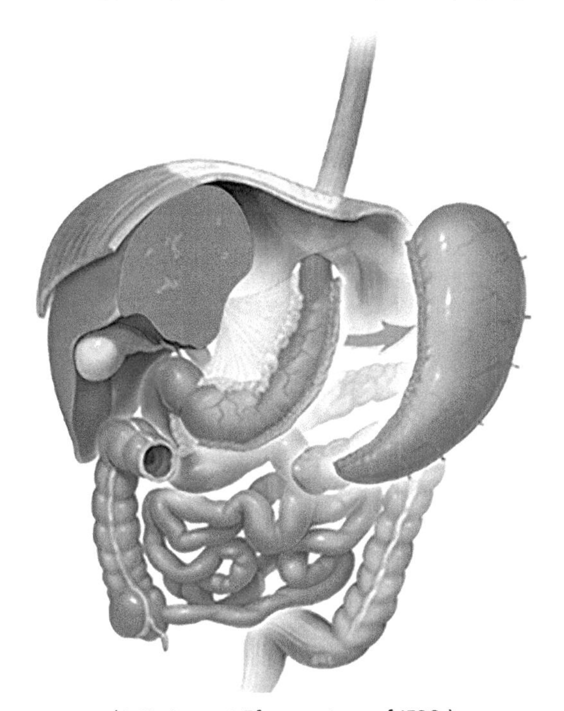

Fig. 2. Sleeve gastrectomy. (© Dr Levent Efe, courtesy of IFSO.)

The most common reoperation after SG is likely for GERD symptoms. It must be emphasized that reported GERD symptoms without confirmatory objective tests such as pH-metry, or the presence of esophagitis is an unreliable predictor of actual GERD. As many reports indicate the improvement of GERD symptoms after a variety of interventions, their validity is suspect without proper objective evidence of GERD. However, as GERD is primarily a quality of life (QOL) issue, symptomatic improvement can be just as important as properly diagnosing the disease. However, as interventions are required, the ethics of this rationale is questionable.

The combination of creating a high-pressure gastric tube, disturbing the angle of His and sling fibers makes the LES function and hiatus more important to prevent reflux. Restoration of the normal hiatus with reduction and fixation of the LES below the hiatus can help prevent reflux. Magnetic sphincter augmentation, likewise, should be of benefit, even if experience is lacking. Conversion to GBP is not always curative of these symptoms, especially in the presence of esophageal motility issues. This underscores the importance of preoperative evaluation, similar to the workup before elective Nissen fundoplication.

It is interesting how often hiatal hernias are observed following bariatric surgery. Although obesity, itself, is a risk for hiatal hernia and GERD, why would there be a higher prevalence after surgery? This concept is not universally accepted, but reports of "pouch migration" and our observation through video archiving every case demonstrating de novo hiatal hernia formation.[23]

The biochemical postprandial changes that occur after SG ironically similar to that of the GBP. This would explain the underwhelming response of the patient to conversion to GBP for weight loss alone. As stated before, the initial response of the patient to any intervention can help predict their response to a similar intervention, in this case GBP. Therefore, consideration should be for a more potent procedure, single-anastomosis duodenal ileostomy (SADI), duodenal switch (DS), or one-anastomosis gastric bypass (OAGB). As a rule, the more intestine bypassed, the more nutritional concerns. This is the case here as well. Consideration for patient compliance with vitamin supplementation and follow-up must be regarded in this context.

It is clear that several SG patients should not be considered conversions but as staged procedures. In the patients with high BMI or central obesity, the risks of primary operative DS or SADI are inherently greater than SG alone; therefore, surgeons will often choose to perform only the SG with the intent on performing a SADI or DS after significant weight loss. An undefinable number of patients will do very well with the SG and not need an intestinal bypass to obtain results. Also, in the time from primary to secondary procedure, one can evaluate the compliance and psychosocial impact of the primary procedure, thus an important factor to consider before committing to further more complex procedures.

ROUX-EN-Y GASTRIC BYPASS

Although the RYGB has been the "gold-standard" operation for comparison purposes, its basic anatomic construct has undergone incremental changes over time, especially since the revolution from open to laparoscopic surgery. No longer thought of as a combined "restrictive/malabsorptive" procedure, the concept of maximizing performance by reducing the size of the gastric pouch/anastomosis and/or increasing the Roux limb length has shown short-term success, but it is unclear by what mechanism this occurs. Hamdi reported a BMI reduction of 8 points at 1 year, but at 2 years increased by 3 points.[24] Dolan reported an average of 15 kg weight loss 5 years after surgical or endoscopic GJ reduction.[25] Placing a prosthetic band or ring, even AGB have reportedly good success rates, but complications such as erosion or intolerance due to dysphagia or reflux remain a concern (**Fig. 3**).[26,27]

Reducing the total alimentary limb length (distalization type: 1) has an effect on improved glycemic control and weight loss, as opposed to shortening the common channel only (distalization type: 2), which has little effect. The effect on weight loss is variable, especially in individuals with BMIs more than 50 kg/m^2.[28]

Conversion of RYGBP to DS or SADI requires taking down the gastrojejunostomy, re-anastomosing the gastric pouch to the remnant stomach as such as was to create an anatomically correct SG without causing injury to the vagus nerves. In our experience, with meticulous reconstruction, the failure rate is too high to risk a single stage due to ischemia of the tissue. Therefore, this is often a multistage operation, and still there is risk of reflux and GERD symptoms due to delayed gastric emptying and/or bile reflux.

Kermansaravi performed a systematic review and meta-analysis of revision procedures after GBP for weight regain. This illustrates the problem with lack of standardized reporting metrics and sporadic follow-up.[29] There has been a tendency to move more toward limb modifications, that is, shortening the total alimentary length with increasing the biliopancreatic limb (distalization type: 1) in primary patients for better metabolic performance. However, as Nimeri points out, without measuring total bowel length on every patient, our data will always be incomplete (**Fig. 4**).[30]

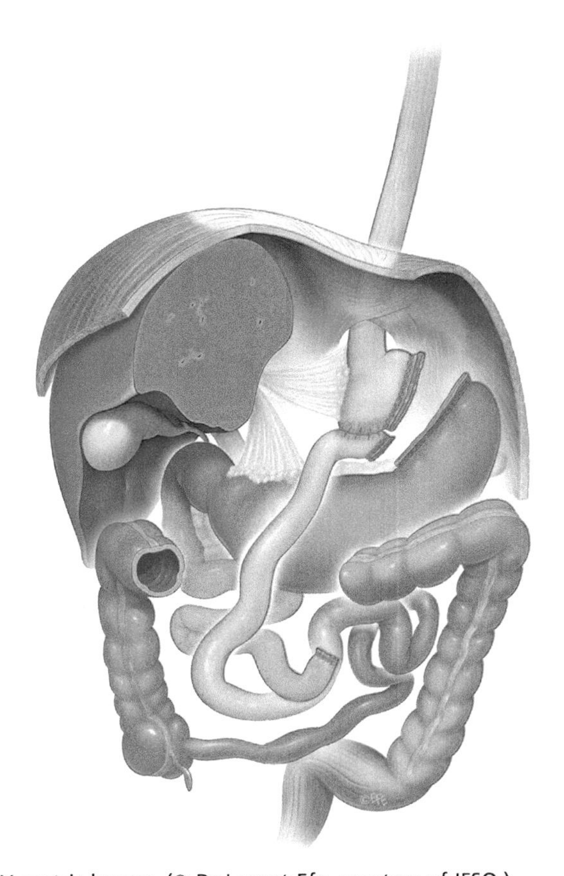

Fig. 3. Roux-en-Y gastric bypass. (© Dr Levent Efe, courtesy of IFSO.)

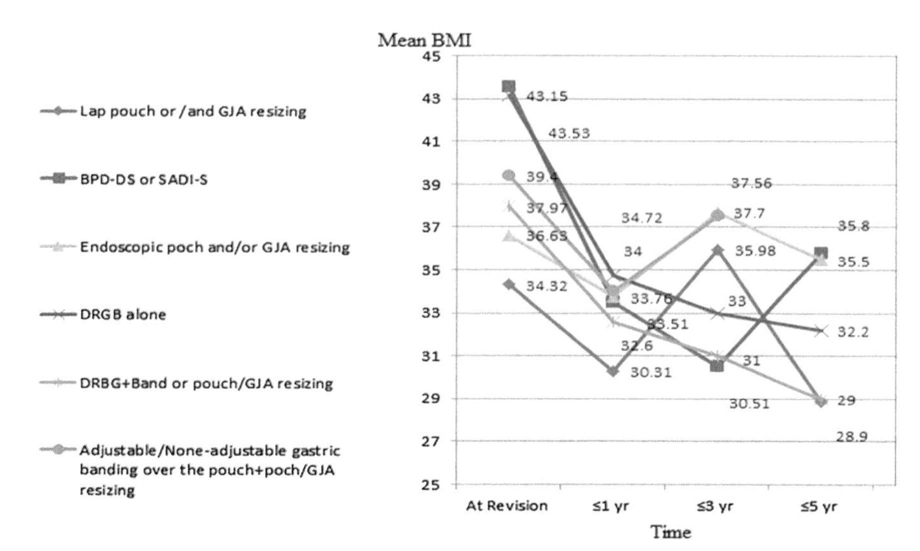

Fig. 4. Effect of different revision surgeries on BMI. *BMI* body mass index, BPD-DS biliopancreatic diversion with duodenal switch, *SADI-S* single-anastomosis duodeno-ileal anastomosis. (*From* Kermansaravi et al.[23])

SINGLE-ANASTOMOSIS DUODENAL ILEOSTOMY AND DUODENAL SWITCH

For weight regain or inadequate weight loss, the SADI can be converted to Roux-en-Y DS by dividing the biliopancreatic limb at the duodenal ileostomy and connecting further downstream, thus diverting bile and pancreatic fluid from mixing with ingested nutrients until about a meter from the ileocecal valve. Both the SADI and DS may also

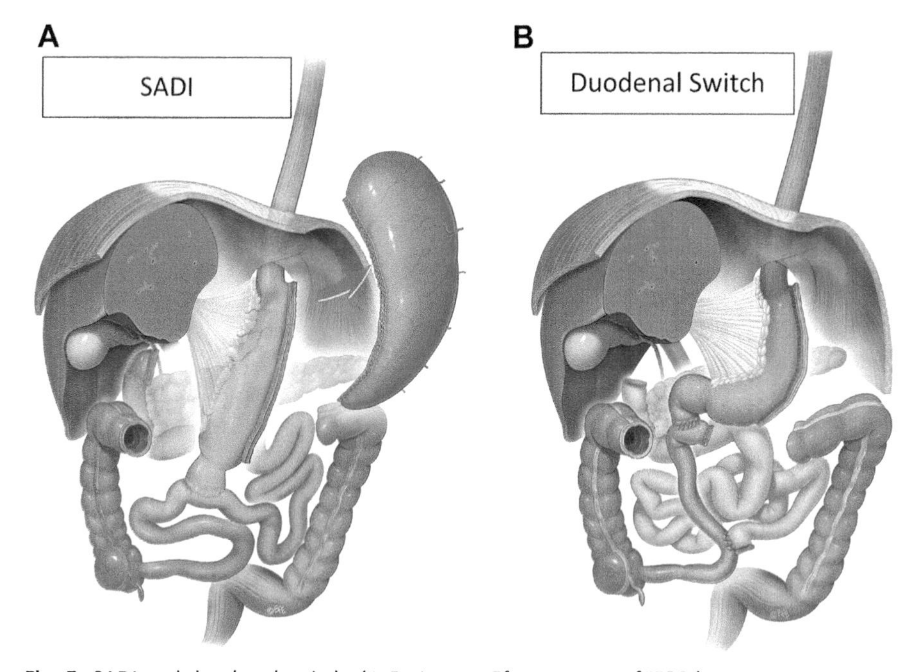

Fig. 5. SADI and duodenal switch. (© Dr Levent Efe, courtesy of IFSO.)

benefit from downsizing the SG further, but there is very little reported experience with these modifications. It was once proposed that the DS should have a larger sleeve for fear of protein–calorie malnutrition, but in patients with inadequate weight loss, this is not a concern. The DS is considered the most aggressive metabolic procedure, and further modifications are entirely investigational (**Fig. 5**).

SUMMARY

There is no debate that metabolic/bariatric surgery is safe and effective.[31] Perioperative complication management requires early recognition and a multidisciplinary approach for best outcomes. Unique to this patient population, long-term complications and weight regain also need to be addressed in the context of a chronic disease model.[32]

DISCLOSURE

None.

REFERENCES

1. American Society for Metabolic and Bariatric Surgery Clinical Issues Committee ASMBS updated position statement on prophy- lactic measures to reduce the risk of venous thromboembolism in bariatric surgery patients. Surg Obes Relat Dis 2013;9(4):493–7.
2. Shaheen O, Siejka J, Thatigotla B, et al. A systematic review of portomesenteric vein thrombosis after sleeve gastrectomy. Surg Obes Relat Dis 2017;13: 1422–31.
3. Godoroja-Diarto Daniela, Copaescu Catalin, Rusu Elena, et al. The role of thromboprophylaxis in patients with portal vein thrombosis: a life-threatening complication after laparoscopic sleeve gastrectomy following 8 years of experience in a bariatric center of excellence. Diagnostics 2022;13(1):43.
4. Gero D, Raptis DA, Vleeschouwers W, et al. Defining global benchmarks in bariatric surgery: a retrospective multicenter analysis of minimally invasive roux-en-y gastric bypass and sleeve gastrectomy. Ann Surg 2019;270(5):859–67.
5. Kassir Radwan, Debs Tarek, Blanc Pierre, Gugenheim Jean, Imed Ben Amor, Boutet Claire, Olivier Tiffet. Complications of bariatric surgery: Presentation and emergency management. Int J Surg 2016;27:77–81.
6. Al-Sabah S, Ladouceur M, Christou N. Anastomotic leaks after bariatric surgery: it is the host response that matters. Surg Obes Relat Dis 2008;4(2):152–7.
7. Manos T, Nedelcu M, Nedelcu A, et al. Leak after sleeve gastrectomy: updated algorithm of treatment. Obes Surg 2021;31(11):4861–7.
8. Rodrigues-Pinto Eduardo, Pereira P, Sousa-pinto B, et al. Retrospective multicenter study on endoscopic treatment of upper GI postsurgical leaks. Gastrointest Endosc 2021;93(6):1283–99.
9. Nimeri AA, Maasher A, Al Shaban T, et al. Internal hernia following laparoscopic roux-en-y gastric bypass: prevention and tips for intra-operative management. Obes Surg 2016;26(9):2255–6.
10. Beran A, Shaear M, Al-Mudares S, et al. Predictors of marginal ulcer after gastric bypass: a systematic review and meta-analysis. J Gastrointestinal Surg 2023. https://doi.org/10.1007/s11605-023-05619-7.

11. Martinino A, Bhandari M, Abouelazayem M, et al. Perforated marginal ulcer after gastric bypass for obesity: a systematic review. Surg Obes Relat Dis 2022;18(9): 1168–75. J Gastrointest Surg. 2023 Feb 16.
12. Ma P, Ghiassi S, Lloyd A, et al. Reversal of Roux en Y gastric bypass: largest single institution experience. Surg Obes Relat Dis 2019 Aug;15(8):1311–6.
13. Dib VRM, Madalosso CAS, Scortegagna GT, et al. Conversion of Roux-en-Y gastric bypass to single anastomosis duodenal ileal bypass with sleeve gastrectomy with gastrogastric jejunal bridge. MethodsX 2022;10:101971.
14. Fecso AB, Di Palma A, Maeda A, et al. Operative management of recalcitrant marginal ulcers following laparoscopic Roux-en-Y gastric bypass for morbid obesity: a systematic review. Surg Obes Relat Dis 2021;17(12):2082–90.
15. Salehi M, Vella A, McLaughlin T, et al. Hypoglycemia after gastric bypass surgery: current concepts and controversies. J Clin Endocrinol Metab 2018; 103(8):2815–26.
16. Byrne TK. Complications of surgery for obesity. Surg Clin North Am 2001;81: 1181–93.
17. Courcoulas AP, King WC, Belle SH, et al. Seven-year weight trajectories and health outcomes in the longitudinal assessment of bariatric surgery (LABS) study. JAMA Surg 2018;153(5):427–34.
18. Kurian M, Sultan S, Garg K, et al. Evaluating gastric erosion in band management: an algorithm for stratification of risk. Surg Obes Relat Dis 2010;6(4): 386–9.
19. Peterli R, Wölnerhanssen BK, Peters T, et al. Prospective study of a two-stage operative concept in the treatment of morbid obesity: primary lap-band® followed if needed by sleeve gastrectomy with duodenal switch. Obes Surg 2007;17(3):334–40.
20. Eisenberg D, Shikora SA, Aarts E, et al. American Society for Metabolic and Bariatric Surgery (ASMBS) and International Federation for the surgery of obesity and metabolic disorders (IFSO): indications for metabolic and bariatric surgery. Surg Obes Relat Dis 2022;18(12):1345–56.
21. Nevo N, Abu-Abeid S, Lahat G, et al. Converting a sleeve gastrectomy to a gastric bypass for weight loss failure—is it worth it? Obes Surg 2018;28(2):364–8.
22. Franken RJ, Sluiter NR, Franken J, et al. Treatment options for weight regain or insufficient weight loss after sleeve gastrectomy: a systematic review and meta-analysis. Obes Surg 2022;32(6):2035–46.
23. Arnoldner MA, Felsenreich DM, Langer FB, et al. Pouch volume and pouch migration after Roux-en-Y gastric bypass: a comparison of gastroscopy and 3 D-CT volumetry: is there a "migration crisis. Surg Obes Relat Dis 2020;16(12): 1902–8.
24. Hamdi A, Julien C, Brown P, et al. Midterm outcomes of revisional surgery for gastric pouch and gastrojejunal anastomotic enlargement in patients with weight regain after gastric bypass for morbid obesity. Obes Surg 2014;24: 1386–90.
25. Dolan RD, Jirapinyo P, Thompson CC. Endoscopic versus surgical gastrojejunal revision for weight regain in Roux-en-Y gastric bypass patients: 5-year safety and efficacy comparison. Gastrointest Endosc 2021;94(5):945–50.
26. Vijgen GH, Schouten R, Bouvy ND, et al. Salvage banding for failed Roux-en-Y gastric bypass. Surg Obes Relat Dis 2012;8(6):803–8.
27. Schmidt HJ, Lee EW, Amianda EA, et al. Large series examining laparoscopic adjustable gastric banding as a salvage solution for failed gastric bypass. Surg Obes Relat Dis 2018;14(12):1869–75.

28. Ghiassi S, Higa K, Chang S, et al. Conversion of standard Roux-en-Y gastric bypass to distal bypass for weight loss failure and metabolic syndrome: 3-year follow-up and evolution of technique to reduce nutritional complications. Surg Obes Relat Dis 2018;14(5):554–61.
29. Kermansaravi M, Davarpanah Jazi AH, Shahabi Shahmiri S, et al. Revision procedures after initial Roux-en-Y gastric bypass, treatment of weight regain: a systematic review and meta-analysis. Updates Surg 2021;73(2):663–78.
30. Wang A, Poliakin L, Sundaresan N, et al. The role of total alimentary limb length in Roux-en-Y gastric bypass: a systematic review. Surg Obes Relat Dis 2022;18(4):555–63.
31. Arterburn DE, Telem DA, Kushner RF, et al. Benefits and risks of bariatric surgery in adults: a review. JAMA 2020;324(9):879–87.
32. Pournaras DJ, Welbourn R. Chronic disease model of shared care after obesity and metabolic surgery. Obes Surg 2018;28(1):255–6.

Endoscopic Management of Surgical Complications of Bariatric Surgery

Khushboo Gala, MBBS, Vitor Brunaldi, MD, PhD,
Barham K. Abu Dayyeh, MD, MPH*

KEYWORDS

- Bariatric surgery • Complications • Endoscopy • Minimally invasive

KEY POINTS

- Upper endoscopy is one of the most important diagnostic tools for complications of bariatric surgery.
- Endoscopic tools and techniques have also revolutionized the management of these complications. These include hemostatic techniques and clips, tissue sealants, endoscopic suturing (such as the FDA-approved Apollo OverStitch system), endoscopic stents (partially or fully covered self-expanding metallic stents or lumen apposing metal stents), and endoscopic vacuum therapy.
- Given their high success rates and low adverse effects, endoscopic modalities are an attractive option for the management for these complications.

INTRODUCTION

The incidence of obesity continues to rise alarmingly, with the current prevalence of obesity in the United States at a staggering 42.4% in 2018.[1] There is also an associated increase in the incidence of obesity-related conditions including heart disease, stroke, type 2 diabetes, and certain types of cancer. Bariatric surgery is the only effective treatment for severe obesity and associated co-morbidities. Roux-en-Y gastric bypass (RYGB) and laparoscopic sleeve gastrectomy (LSG) are both effective procedures for weight loss and currently comprise more than 75% of performed procedures.[2] RYGB is currently the most effective treatment for obesity, with maximal weight loss of around 30% total body weight loss seen within the first 1 to 2 years, and long-term data showing that patients with

Department of Gastroenterology and Hepatology, Mayo Clinic, 200 First Street South West, Rochester, MN 55905, USA
* Corresponding author.
E-mail address: abudayyeh.barham@mayo.edu

Gastroenterol Clin N Am 52 (2023) 719–731
https://doi.org/10.1016/j.gtc.2023.08.004

RYGB are able to maintain more than 25% of total weight loss even over 20 years.[3] In general, bariatric procedures are also preferred in patients with obesity-related co-morbidities like type 2 diabetes mellitus, nonalcoholic fatty liver disease, metabolic syndrome, and polycystic ovarian syndrome. However, bariatric surgery is not exempt from complications, especially given the complex surgical anatomy with multiple staple lines and anastomoses. Additionally, the remnant stomach continues to remain physiologically active in RYGB, leading to a potential further risk of chronic complications. The complication rate after bariatric surgery is approximately 15%, although most are minor.[4] The most common ones are marginal ulcers, anastomotic strictures and leaks, gastrogastric fistulas (GGFs), dumping syndrome, gastroesophageal reflux disease, and weight regain. There are several endoscopic tools available in practice today that serve as invaluable and often first-line resources to manage those complications. Commonly used tools are conventional endoscopic techniques like hemostatic techniques and clips, tissue sealants, endoscopic suturing (such as the Food and Drug Administration-approved Apollo OverStitch system), endoscopic stents (partially or fully covered self-expanding metallic stents [SEMSs] or lumen apposing metal stents [LAMSs]), and endoscopic vacuum therapy (EVT). This review will provide a comprehensive overview of the techniques and devices to address the most frequent postoperative complications.

Marginal Ulceration (Roux-en-Y Gastric Bypass)

Ulceration seen at the gastrojejunal anastomosis (GJA), termed as marginal ulceration, is a common complication seen after bariatric surgery, with a reported incidence of 3% to 7%.[5] Marginal ulcers have a multifactorial pathophysiology, with different contributory factors for early and late ulceration. Local factors like inflammation and technical aspects of anastomosis creation lend a part in early ulceration, while microvascular ischemia plays a major role in late ulceration.[6] A study looking at Nationwide Inpatient Sample data from 2003 to 2011 found the most prominent risk factor to be chronic nonsteroidal anti-inflammatory drug (NSAID) use.[7] Other purported risk factors include *Helicobacter pylori* infection, diabetes mellitus, obstructive sleep apnea, female sex, smoking, and alcohol dependence.

Most marginal ulcers respond to medical management with antisecretory agents and cessation of smoking and NSAID use. The use of high-dose proton pump inhibitors twice daily in an open capsule protocol, along with sucralfate, has been shown to be useful.[6] A minority of patients (<10%) may have persistent symptoms despite medical management, including intractable pain and recurrent gastrointestinal hemorrhage. In these cases, endoscopic therapies are a useful adjunct to surgical revision.

Endoscopy is a valuable tool to confirm the diagnosis of marginal ulcers and carefully examine the ulcer bed for the presence of sutures and foreign objects. Evaluation for a GGF is also key in cases of refractory ulceration. The presence of nonabsorbable sutures serves as an irritant to the gastric mucosa and promotes nonhealing of the marginal ulcer. These can be removed using tools like biopsy forceps, endoscopic scissors (cuts silk sutures), and loop cutters (cuts Prolene sutures), and rat-tooth forceps (removes staple chains).[8,9] In cases of bleeding ulcers, standard endoscopic management with mechanical hemostasis (such as clipping) and epinephrine injection is recommended. In cases with refractory bleeding or recalcitrant ulcers, there are emerging data on oversewing of ulcers using endoscopic suturing systems.[10–12] Lastly, endoscopic reversal of RYGB anatomy has also been described, which is particularly valuable in patients with recalcitrant ulcers who are poor surgical candidates. This is performed by creating an endoscopic ultrasound-guided GGF, followed by using an endoscopic suturing system to close the gastrojejunostomy stoma.[13]

Anastomotic Strictures (Roux-en-Y Gastric Bypass)

Anastomotic strictures or stenoses are most commonly seen at the GJA, with a reported incidence of 0.3% to 0.5%.[14] Causes entail ischemia, tension on the anastomosis, edema, or a foreign-body reaction. Risk factors for strictures include old age, circular stapled gastrojejunostomy, and postoperative complications like anastomotic leaks, fistulas, and marginal ulceration.[15] Strictures are generally symptomatic when they narrow to a diameter of less than 10 mm.[16]

As with other complications, endoscopy is a valuable tool for the diagnosis of anastomotic strictures. The first line for management of strictures is endoscopic dilation. This is a safe and highly effective technique, with reported success rates of higher than 95%.[17,18] A large ischemic segment and the presence of a fistula were found to be risk factors for failure of dilation. The timing of dilation after RYGB may also play a role, with 1 study showing that dilation may be less effective if performed more than 90 days after surgery.[19] Dilation can be performed with both hydrostatic balloon and mechanical Savary-Gilliard bougies, although through-the-scope (TTS) endoscopic balloon dilation is the more popular choice. To decrease the risk of perforation, strictures should not be dilated by more than 3 to 4 mm at a time.[20] Strictures should generally be dilated to 12 to 15 mm, keeping in mind that overdilation may reduce the restrictive effect of RYGB.[21] As a result, serial dilations are often required, with a mean of 2 dilations required for optimal dilation seen in a large retrospective analysis.[22] Complications of endoscopic dilation include bleeding and perforation. The risk of perforation is low, yet not insignificant at 0% to 3%, with an increased risk of perforation with greater number of dilation sessions.[14,17]

A small fraction of strictures can be refractory to standard dilation therapy. One option is using intramucosal steroids (triamcinolone acetonide) immediately after balloon dilation.[23–26] Needle knife can also be used to open more fibrotic or obstructed strictures.[23,27] Using SEMSs or LAMSs is another option to manage refractory strictures. SEMSs have been used traditionally with variable results; however, they are associated with a risk of stent migration, tissue ingrowth, and stent intolerance.[28] There is a growing pool of data supporting the use of LAMS for stenting.[29–32] SEMSs have a higher rate of adverse effects, which may be lower in LAMSs given their smaller and dumbbell-shaped configuration.[33,34] One study showed that migrated LAMSs generally pass spontaneously, without requiring endoscopic or laparoscopic removal.[29] Securing the stent in place using endoscopic suturing might help decrease the risk of migration, however, this adds to the complexity and length of the procedure. This technique has been studied with both SEMS and LAMS, with a migration rate of 0% seen with LAMS.[35,36] In general, stents should be removed or exchanged after 3 to 6 months due to the risk of stent breakdown and migration. With multiple therapeutic options available endoscopically, the need for surgical revision of anastomotic strictures is extremely uncommon.

Anastomotic/Staple Line Leaks (Roux-en-Y Gastric Bypass/Laparoscopic Sleeve Gastrectomy)

Anastomotic or staple line leaks (ASL) are rare but dreaded complications of RYGB and LSG, respectively, with a reported incidence of 0.5% to 5% and a lower incidence seen with more experienced surgeons.[37] They are most frequently seen at the GJA and after revisional RYGB surgery. Endoscopy can help with both diagnosis and management of ASL.

Diagnosis of ASL can be challenging, as clinical findings are varied and can often be subtle in patients with severe obesity. Using air inflation during intraoperative endoscopy can help detect early leaks and facilitate intraoperative repair.[15] However, retrospective data analyzing the impact of intraoperative leak testing have not yielded significant results.[38]

Management of leaks is dependent on the clinical stability of the patient, the chronicity of the leak, and the presence of organized fluid collections. If an acute leak is suspected clinically and the patient is unstable with systemic inflammatory response syndrome or peritonitis, surgical exploration should be prioritized. In this setting, simultaneous endoscopic placement of stents is useful.[39] For more stable patients, endoscopic repair techniques can be an option. Endoscopic repair strategies can be divided into techniques for wall closure, diversion of contents, and endoscopic internal drainage (EID) of fluid collections. EID is generally accomplished using pigtail catheters draining into the collection or EVT. This involves the placement of an intraluminal or extraluminal sponge or covered gauze with an externalized tube with continuous negative pressure, which helps remove secretion and promote tissue granulation.

Direct wall closure can be attempted if the defect is small and there is no attached fluid collection. Available options include TTS and over-the-scope clips (OTSCs), fibrin glue, and endoluminal suturing devices. The OTSC system has the advantage of being able to close larger defects with greater stability and lesser strain on the surrounding tissue than TTS clips. A review looking at the OTSC system demonstrated good closure rates, with the highest probability of success in patients with small leaks or fistulas and a short interval between diagnosis and intervention.[40] However, the paradigm of management is moving from the use of closure techniques to EVT or EID. This was demonstrated in a recent international multicenter expert survey which showed that the most popular therapeutic option for post-bariatric leaks was a combination of EVT and EID.[41] Still, half of the responders reported using fully covered self-expandable metal stents as their standard first option, mostly associated with techniques to minimize migration.

Use of endoscopic stents is the standard modality used for wall exclusion. Long-term data show a high success rate, a good side-effect profile, and no interference in weight loss.[42] However, a study comparing the use of stents and endoscopic drainage showed that the primary success of stents is inferior to EID (63% vs 86%).[43] In this study, it was notable that patients who failed closure with stent placement had a significant increase in healing with EID. Such modality with the use of double pigtail stents has been shown to be effective and safe. A large cohort of 617 patients undergoing EID showed a clinical success rate of around 85%.[43,44] Concurrent endoscopic necrosectomy and management of downstream stenosis with dilation can also be performed to enhance the success of EID.[39]

Increasingly, EVT is being used in large and complicated leaks with high success rates and minimal adverse effects.[45,46] A recent study comparing EID and EVT showed higher rates of success for EID, but a significantly shorter duration of treatment for EVT. Still, EVT requires a higher number of procedures to achieve success, since the tube needs replacement every few days.[47] In general, each leak should be managed individually, and multiple therapies should be used either concurrently or sequentially before declaring endoscopic failure.[48]

Gastrogastric Fistula (Roux-en-Y Gastric Bypass)

A GGF is an abnormal communication between the gastric pouch and the gastric remnant in RYGB patients. This allows ingested food to enter the bypassed foregut (stomach and duodenum). Consequently, it is 1 of the important causes of weight regain in postsurgical patients. Patients can also suffer from intractable marginal ulceration from acid reflux through the fistula, leading to recurrent gastrointestinal hemorrhage or pain. With contemporary techniques of RYGB surgery, the formation of GGF is rare, with an incidence of 1% to 3%.[49]

Although multiple endoscopic methods have been trialed for management, the ongoing chronic inflammation and ischemia surrounding a GGF make long-term success with endoscopic repair challenging. However, endoscopic strategies can be useful in small fistulas or early cases. The use of argon plasma coagulation and other techniques to debride surrounding mucosa may assist in making endoscopic techniques more effective in closing the GGF.

Endoscopic repair using endoclips can be an option in very small fistulas in select cases.[50,51] In some instances, using a tissue sealant like fibrin glue and cyanoacrylate to close small fistulas has also been described, but may require several reapplications.[52,53] Endoscopic suturing of larger fistulas has also been reported as a technically feasible procedure.[54–56] Although immediate closure is generally successful, this is generally not a viable long-term solution because of high rates of fistula recurrence, described as upwards of 80% at 1 year. Sequential closure in cases with initial failure has mixed results in literature but may be considered in selected high-surgical risk cases.[57,58] Endoscopic stenting of the gastrojejunostomy can be used in early cases.[59,60] Case reports have described the use of cardiac septal defect occluders for endoscopic obliteration of GGF.[61] This needs to be explored further before being used widely in practice. Ultimately, for large, nonhealing, or highly symptomatic fistulas, surgical repair in the form of laparoscopic fistula excision with or without revision of GJA remains the definitive therapy.[62]

Dumping Syndrome (Generally in Roux-en-Y Gastric Bypass)

Early and late dumping syndrome can be seen after RYGB and less commonly with LSG. Early dumping is primarily an osmotic process due to the passage of undigested food into the small intestine triggering rapid fluid shifts into the intestinal lumen. It happens within an hour of eating. Late dumping, also known as postprandial hyperinsulinemic hypoglycemia, has a complex pathophysiology that is not completely understood but includes alterations in multiple hormonal and glycemic patterns. This is much less common, occurring in less than 0.5% of cases,[63] and the onset of symptoms initiates 1 to 3 hours after meals.

The initial management of early and late dumping syndrome is similar and involves dietary modifications, including multiple small meals throughout the day, with foods that are high in fiber and protein, and low in simple carbohydrates. In some cases, medications like nifedipine, acarbose, diazoxide, and octreotide can be useful adjuncts. Glucagon-like peptide-1 receptor blockade also reverses postprandial hypoglycemia and associated autonomic and neuroglycopenic symptoms and can be considered in these cases. There are emerging data on endoscopic management for refractory cases. This involves reducing the diameter of a dilated and incompetent GJA with an endoscopic suturing system (endoscopic transoral outlet reduction [TORe]) (**Fig. 1**). Consequently, there is delayed emptying of the gastric pouch leading to decreased dumping syndrome. A large, multicentric study from our group showed a

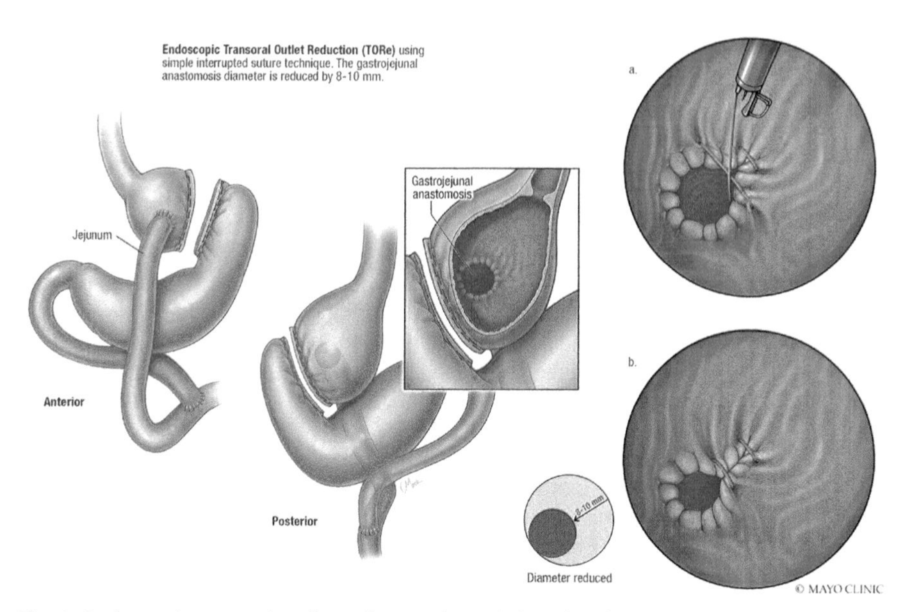

Fig. 1. Endoscopic tansoral outlet reduction (TORe). (Used with permission of Mayo Foundation for Medical Education and Research, all rights reserved.)

high rate of success (>95%) with the use of TORe, with a very low rate of weight regain.[64] In a minority of cases, repeat revision may be required to sustain the clinical resolution.[65] A recent meta-analysis showed a pooled technical success and clinical success rate of 98.15% (94.39%–99.4%) and 89.5% (79.17%–95.03%), respectively.[66] Overall, endoscopic revision seems to be a safe and effective therapy for refractory dumping syndrome and should be explored in all cases prior to surgical revision.

Gastric Stenosis/Twist (Laparoscopic Sleeve Gastrectomy)

Gastric stenosis has been reported in up to 0.7% to 4% of patients after an LSG.[67] It occurs mainly due to a rotation of the staple line and scarring of the sleeve asymmetrically, leading to kinking of the gastric sleeve. Stenosis can be organic with evident luminal narrowing, functional if only a deformation is seen, or have both components. Diagnosis can be challenging, especially in cases with functional stenosis only. Endoscopy may reveal persistently wide-open gastroesophageal junction, dilated upstream stomach, and luminal compromise at the stenosed site. Erosive esophagitis is also frequently associated. Fluoroscopy or an upper gastrointestinal series may be needed to diagnose functional stenosis that is not obviously identified on endoscopy. There are emerging data on the use of endoluminal functional impedance planimetry both for diagnosis and prognostication of sleeve stenosis (**Fig. 2**).[68,69] Patients who are likely to respond to pneumatic dilation have larger mean post-dilation diameter and distensibility index.

Many options have been described for endoscopic management of sleeve stenosis. Balloon dilation is the most commonly performed, with 2 techniques described in the literature—TTS hydrostatic controlled radial expansion balloon and pneumatic balloon (**Fig. 3**).[70,71] With a hydrostatic balloon, the balloon dilation diameter ranges from 10 to 20 mm; compared to this, pneumatic dilation targets a balloon diameter of 30 mm to achieve 18 to 20 psi titrated over 2 minutes under fluoroscopic and

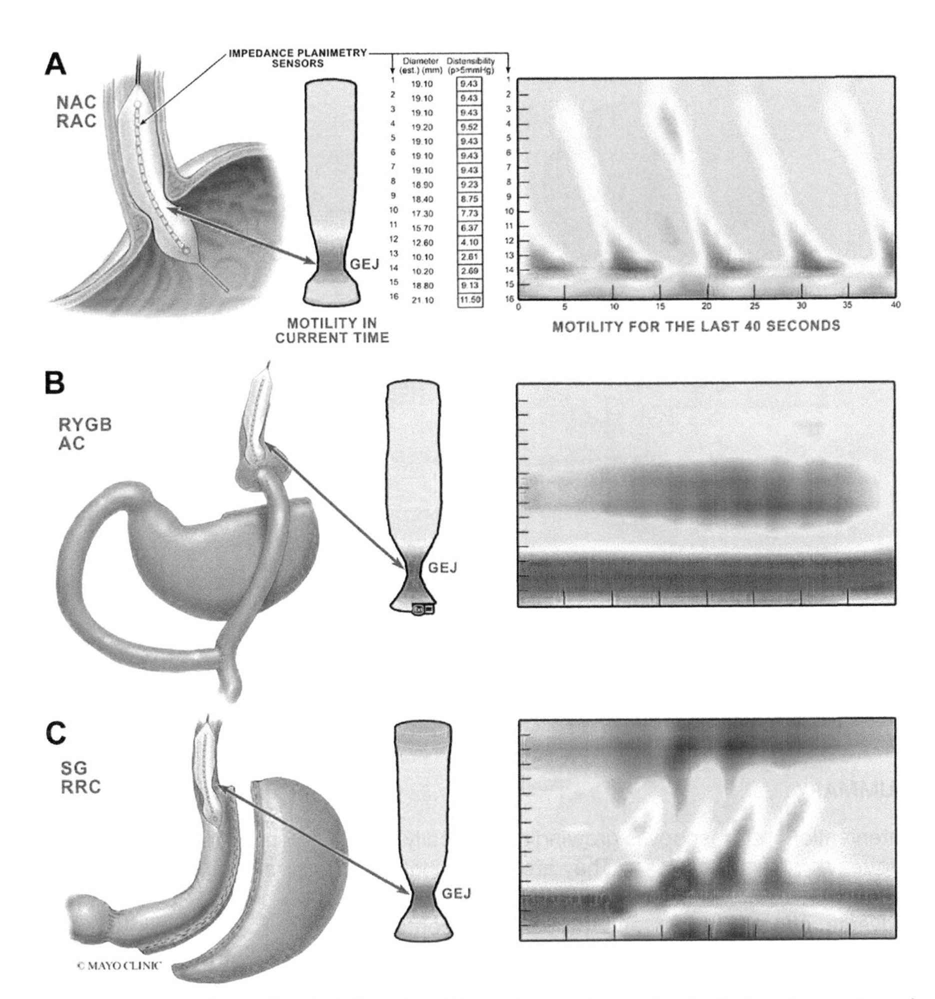

Fig. 2. The use of endoluminal functional impedance planimetry both for diagnosis and prognostication of sleeve stenosis. (Used with permission of Mayo Foundation for Medical Education and Research, all rights reserved.)

endoscopic guidance, with repeat dilations to 35 mm if the initial treatment was unsuccessful. The pneumatic balloon generally provides wider and more forceful dilation and has been shown to have a high rate of success, even greater than 85% in 1 study.[67] Adverse events include perforation; however, this is extremely uncommon. Usually, follow-up dilation sessions are warranted, generally every 2 weeks for up to 4 sessions. A complete helix stricture has been associated with higher rates of failure of therapy. This is a function of the angle within the twist, as well as the presence of a persistently dilated gastric pouch above the kinking.[72] Endoscopic stenting using fully covered stents has also been shown to be a successful modality. The risk of stent migration can be decreased by securing it in place by endoscopic suturing.[73,74] A review proposed using balloon dilation as the first line for management of sleeve stenosis, with use of stenting in refractory cases.[74] Cases that do not respond to endoscopic measures must be referred for surgical evaluation and repair, and possibly conversion to RYGB.[75]

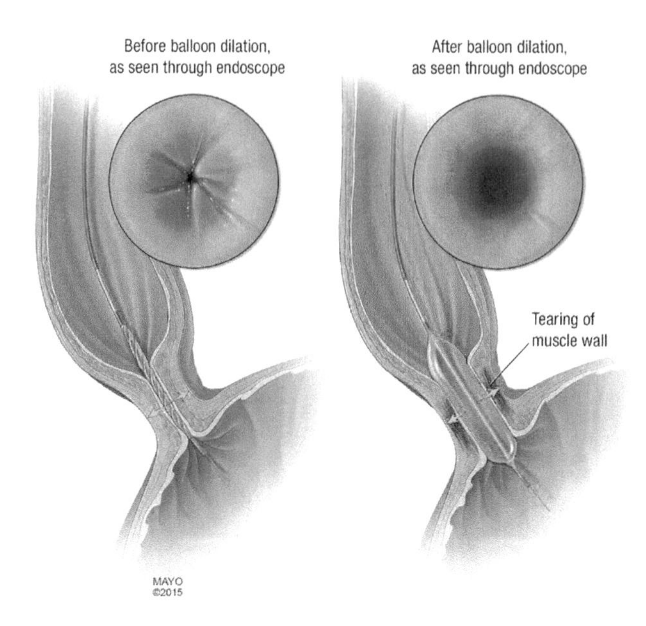

Fig. 3. Pneumatic balloon dilation of gastric stenosis. (Used with permission of Mayo Foundation for Medical Education and Research, all rights reserved.)

SUMMARY

Interventional endoscopy is growing meteorically as a field, with many tools and techniques now at our disposal. They are increasingly the preferred first method of management for complications of bariatric surgery, given high success rates and low adverse effects. Larger and randomized controlled studies are needed to form evidence-based recommendations and guidelines for the use of endoscopic techniques for the management of complications of bariatric surgery and weight regain.

CLINICS CARE POINTS

- Endoscopic oversewing can be a valuable tool in the management of refractory marginal ulceration.
- Endoscopic dilation or lumen apposing metal stents can be used in the management of anastomotic strictures.
- A variety of therapeutic options including clip closure, stents, and endoscopic vacuum therapy can be used for the management of anastomotic leaks.

DISCLOSURE

B.K. Abu Dayyeh Consulting for Endogenex, Endo-TAGSS, Metamodix, and BFKW; consultant and grant/research support from USGI, Apollo Endosurgery, Medtronic, Spatz Medical, EndoGastric Solutions, Aspire Bariatrics, Boston Scientific, United States; Speaker roles with Olympus, Johnson and Johnson; and research support from Cairn Diagnostics, GI Dynamics. Other authors have no relevant disclosures. There were no funding sources for this manuscript.

REFERENCES

1. National Center for Health S, editor. National health and nutrition examination survey 2017–march 2020 prepandemic data files development of files and prevalence estimates for selected health outcomes. Hyattsville, MD: National Health Statistics Reports; 2021.
2. English WJ, DeMaria EJ, Brethauer SA, et al. American Society for Metabolic and Bariatric Surgery estimation of metabolic and bariatric procedures performed in the United States in 2016. Surg Obes Relat Dis 2018;14(3):259–63 [published Online First: 2018/01/27].
3. Sjostrom L. Review of the key results from the Swedish Obese Subjects (SOS) trial - a prospective controlled intervention study of bariatric surgery. J Intern Med 2013;273(3):219–34 [published Online First: 2012/11/21].
4. DeMaria EJ, Pate V, Warthen M, et al. Baseline data from american society for metabolic and bariatric surgery-designated bariatric surgery centers of excellence using the bariatric outcomes longitudinal database. Surg Obes Relat Dis 2010;6(4):347–55 [published Online First: 2010/02/24].
5. Rodrigo DC, Jill S, Daniel M, et al. Which Factors Correlate with Marginal Ulcer After Surgery for Obesity? Obes Surg 2020;30(12):4821–7 [published Online First: 2020/09/18].
6. Schulman AR, Chan WW, Devery A, et al. Opened proton pump inhibitor capsules reduce time to healing compared with intact capsules for marginal ulceration following roux-en-Y gastric bypass. Clin Gastroenterol Hepatol 2017;15(4): 494–500 e1 [published Online First: 2016/10/25].
7. Sweeney TE, Morton JM. Metabolic surgery: action via hormonal milieu changes, changes in bile acids or gut microbiota? a summary of the literature. Best Pract Res Clin Gastroenterol 2014;28(4):727–40 [published Online First: 2014/09/10].
8. Storm AC, Thompson CC. Endoscopic treatments following bariatric surgery. Gastrointest Endosc Clin N Am 2017;27(2):233–44 [published Online First: 2017/03/16].
9. Frezza EE, Herbert H, Ford R, et al. Endoscopic suture removal at gastrojejunal anastomosis after Roux-en-Y gastric bypass to prevent marginal ulceration. Surg Obes Relat Dis 2007;3(6):619–22 [published Online First: 2007/11/21].
10. Agarwal A, Benias P, Brewer Gutierrez OI, et al. Endoscopic suturing for management of peptic ulcer-related upper gastrointestinal bleeding: a preliminary experience. Endosc Int Open 2018;6(12):E1439–44 [published Online First: 2018/12/13].
11. Liu S, Kim R. Successful closure with endoscopic suturing of a recalcitrant marginal ulcer despite Roux-en-Y gastric bypass reversion. VideoGIE 2019;4(12): 554–5 [published Online First: 2019/12/18].
12. Barola S, Magnuson T, Schweitzer M, et al. Endoscopic suturing for massively bleeding marginal ulcer 10 days post roux-en-Y gastric bypass. Obes Surg 2017;27(5):1394–6 [published Online First: 2017/03/02].
13. Jaruvongvanich V, Matar R, Maselli DB, et al. Endoscopic reversal of Roux-en-Y anatomy for the treatment of recurrent marginal ulceration. VideoGIE 2020;5(7): 286–8 [published Online First: 2020/07/10].
14. Almby K, Edholm D. Anastomotic strictures after roux-en-y gastric bypass: a cohort study from the scandinavian obesity surgery registry. Obes Surg 2019; 29(1):172–7 [published Online First: 2018/09/13].

15. Valenzuela-Salazar C, Rojano-Rodriguez ME, Romero-Loera S, et al. Intraoperative endoscopy prevents technical defect related leaks in laparoscopic Roux-en-Y gastric bypass: A randomized control trial. Int J Surg 2018;50:17–21 [published Online First: 2017/12/27].
16. Ukleja A, Afonso BB, Pimentel R, et al. Outcome of endoscopic balloon dilation of strictures after laparoscopic gastric bypass. Surg Endosc 2008;22(8):1746–50 [published Online First: 2008/03/19].
17. de Moura EGH, Orso IRB, Aurelio EF, et al. Factors associated with complications or failure of endoscopic balloon dilation of anastomotic stricture secondary to Roux-en-Y gastric bypass surgery. Surg Obes Relat Dis 2016;12(3):582–6 [published Online First: 2016/05/14].
18. Catalano MF, Chua TY, Rudic G. Endoscopic balloon dilation of stomal stenosis following gastric bypass. Obes Surg 2007;17(3):298–303 [published Online First: 2007/06/06].
19. Yimcharoen P, Heneghan H, Chand B, et al. Successful management of gastrojejunal strictures after gastric bypass: is timing important? Surg Obes Relat Dis 2012;8(2):151–7 [published Online First: 2011/03/29].
20. Go MR, Muscarella P 2nd, Needleman BJ, et al. Endoscopic management of stomal stenosis after Roux-en-Y gastric bypass. Surg Endosc 2004;18(1):56–9 [published Online First: 2003/11/20].
21. Peifer KJ, Shiels AJ, Azar R, et al. Successful endoscopic management of gastrojejunal anastomotic strictures after Roux-en-Y gastric bypass. Gastrointest Endosc 2007;66(2):248–52 [published Online First: 2007/04/25].
22. Carrodeguas L, Szomstein S, Zundel N, et al. Gastrojejunal anastomotic strictures following laparoscopic Roux-en-Y gastric bypass surgery: analysis of 1291 patients. Surg Obes Relat Dis 2006;2(2):92–7 [published Online First: 2006/08/24].
23. Larsen M, Kozarek R. Therapeutic endoscopy for the treatment of post-bariatric surgery complications. World J Gastroenterol 2022;28(2):199–215 [published Online First: 2022/02/04].
24. Hanaoka N, Ishihara R, Motoori M, et al. Endoscopic Balloon Dilation Followed By Intralesional Steroid Injection for Anastomotic Strictures After Esophagectomy: A Randomized Controlled Trial. Am J Gastroenterol 2018;113(10):1468–74 [published Online First: 2018/09/06].
25. van der Have M, Noomen C, Oldenburg B, et al. Balloon dilatation with or without intralesional and oral corticosteroids for anastomotic Crohn's disease strictures. J Gastrointestin Liver Dis 2015;24(4):537–9 [published Online First: 2015/12/24].
26. Van Assche G. Intramural steroid injection and endoscopic dilation for Crohn's disease. Clin Gastroenterol Hepatol 2007;5(9):1027–8 [published Online First: 2007/09/11].
27. Lee JK, Van Dam J, Morton JM, et al. Endoscopy is accurate, safe, and effective in the assessment and management of complications following gastric bypass surgery. Am J Gastroenterol 2009;104(3):575–82, quiz 83.
28. Vedantam S, Roberts J. Endoscopic Stents in the Management of Bariatric Complications: Our Algorithm and Outcomes. Obes Surg 2020;30(3):1150–8 [published Online First: 2019/12/01].
29. Skidmore AP. Use of lumen-apposing metal stents (LAMS) in the management of gastro jejunostomy stricture following Roux-en-Y Gastric Bypass for obesity: a prospective series. BMC Surg 2021;21(1):314 [published Online First: 2021/07/19].
30. Bazerbachi F, Heffley JD, Abu Dayyeh BK, et al. Safety and efficacy of coaxial lumen-apposing metal stents in the management of refractory gastrointestinal

luminal strictures: a multicenter study. Endosc Int Open 2017;5(9):E861–7 [published Online First: 2017/09/20].
31. McCarty TR, Kumar N. Revision Bariatric Procedures and Management of Complications from Bariatric Surgery. Dig Dis Sci 2022;67(5):1688–701 [published Online First: 2022/03/30].
32. Sharma P, McCarty TR, Chhoda A, et al. Alternative uses of lumen apposing metal stents. World J Gastroenterol 2020;26(21):2715–28 [published Online First: 2020/06/20].
33. Puig CA, Waked TM, Baron TH, et al. The role of endoscopic stents in the management of chronic anastomotic and staple line leaks and chronic strictures after bariatric surgery. Surg Obes Relat Dis 2014;10(4):613–7 [published Online First: 2014/04/01].
34. Mansoor MS, Tejada J, Parsa NA, et al. Off label use of lumen-apposing metal stent for persistent gastro-jejunal anastomotic stricture. World J Gastrointest Endosc 2018;10(6):117–20 [published Online First: 2018/07/11].
35. Simsek C, Ichkhanian Y, Fayad L, et al. Secured Lumen-Apposing Fully Covered Metallic Stents for Stenoses in Post-Bariatric Surgery Patients. Obes Surg 2019;29(8):2695–9 [published Online First: 2019/05/06].
36. Fayad L, Simsek C, Oleas R, et al. Safety and Efficacy of Endoscopically Secured Fully Covered Self-Expandable Metallic Stents (FCSEMS) for Post-Bariatric Complex Stenosis. Obes Surg 2019;29(11):3484–92 [published Online First: 2019/06/30].
37. Griffith PS, Birch DW, Sharma AM, et al. Managing complications associated with laparoscopic Roux-en-Y gastric bypass for morbid obesity. Can J Surg 2012;55(5):329–36 [published Online First: 2012/08/03].
38. Liu N, Cusack MC, Venkatesh M, et al. 30-Day Outcomes After Intraoperative Leak Testing for Bariatric Surgery Patients. J Surg Res 2019;242:136–44 [published Online First: 2019/05/12].
39. Vargas EJ, Abu Dayyeh BK. Keep calm under pressure: a paradigm shift in managing postsurgical leaks. Gastrointest Endosc 2018;87(2):438–41 [published Online First: 2018/02/07].
40. Shoar S, Poliakin L, Khorgami Z, et al. Efficacy and Safety of the Over-the-Scope Clip (OTSC) System in the Management of Leak and Fistula After Laparoscopic Sleeve Gastrectomy: a Systematic Review. Obes Surg 2017;27(9):2410–8 [published Online First: 2017/03/30].
41. Rodrigues-Pinto E, Repici A, Donatelli G, et al. International multicenter expert survey on endoscopic treatment of upper gastrointestinal anastomotic leaks. Endosc Int Open 2019;7(12):E1671–82 [published Online First: 2019/12/04].
42. Krishnan V, Hutchings K, Godwin A, et al. Long-term outcomes following endoscopic stenting in the management of leaks after foregut and bariatric surgery. Surg Endosc 2019;33(8):2691–5 [published Online First: 2019/02/01].
43. Lorenzo D, Guilbaud T, Gonzalez JM, et al. Endoscopic treatment of fistulas after sleeve gastrectomy: a comparison of internal drainage versus closure. Gastrointest Endosc 2018;87(2):429–37 [published Online First: 2017/07/29].
44. Donatelli G, Spota A, Cereatti F, et al. Endoscopic internal drainage for the management of leak, fistula, and collection after sleeve gastrectomy: our experience in 617 consecutive patients. Surg Obes Relat Dis 2021;17(8):1432–9 [published Online First: 2021/05/02].
45. Hayami M, Klevebro F, Tsekrekos A, et al. Endoscopic vacuum therapy for anastomotic leak after esophagectomy: a single-center's early experience. Dis

Esophagus 2021;34(9). https://doi.org/10.1093/dote/doaa122 [published Online First: 2020/12/29].

46. Rodrigues-Pinto E, Morais R, Vilas-Boas F, et al. Role of endoscopic vacuum therapy, internal drainage, and stents for postbariatric leaks. VideoGIE 2019;4(10):481–5 [published Online First: 2019/11/12].
47. Jung CFM, Hallit R, Muller-Dornieden A, et al. Endoscopic internal drainage and low negative-pressure endoscopic vacuum therapy for anastomotic leaks after oncologic upper gastrointestinal surgery. Endoscopy 2022;54(1):71–4 [published Online First: 2021/01/29].
48. Merrifield BF, Lautz D, Thompson CC. Endoscopic repair of gastric leaks after Roux-en-Y gastric bypass: a less invasive approach. Gastrointest Endosc 2006;63(4):710–4 [published Online First: 2006/03/28].
49. Carrodeguas L, Szomstein S, Soto F, et al. Management of gastrogastric fistulas after divided Roux-en-Y gastric bypass surgery for morbid obesity: analysis of 1,292 consecutive patients and review of literature. Surg Obes Relat Dis 2005;1(5):467–74 [published Online First: 2006/08/24].
50. Bhardwaj A, Cooney RN, Wehrman A, et al. Endoscopic repair of small symptomatic gastrogastric fistulas after gastric bypass surgery: a single center experience. Obes Surg 2010;20(8):1090–5 [published Online First: 2010/05/05].
51. Fernandez-Esparrach G, Lautz DB, Thompson CC. Endoscopic repair of gastrogastric fistula after Roux-en-Y gastric bypass: a less-invasive approach. Surg Obes Relat Dis 2010;6(3):282–8 [published Online First: 2010/06/01].
52. Gumbs AA, Duffy AJ, Bell RL. Management of gastrogastric fistula after laparoscopic Roux-en-Y gastric bypass. Surg Obes Relat Dis 2006;2(2):117–21 [published Online First: 2006/08/24].
53. Rogalski P, Swidnicka-Siergiejko A, Wasielica-Berger J, et al. Endoscopic management of leaks and fistulas after bariatric surgery: a systematic review and meta-analysis. Surg Endosc 2021;35(3):1067–87 [published Online First: 2020/02/29].
54. Tsai C, Kessler U, Steffen R, et al. Endoscopic Closure of Gastro-gastric Fistula After Gastric Bypass: a Technically Feasible Procedure but Associated with Low Success Rate. Obes Surg 2019;29(1):23–7 [published Online First: 2018/09/03].
55. Kumbhari V, le Roux CW, Cohen RV. Endoscopic Evaluation and Management of Late Complications After Bariatric Surgery: a Narrative Review. Obes Surg 2021;31(10):4624–33 [published Online First: 2021/08/01].
56. Zhang LY, Bejjani M, Ghandour B, et al. Endoscopic through-the-scope suturing. VideoGIE 2022;7(1):46–51 [published Online First: 2022/01/22].
57. Mukewar S, Kumar N, Catalano M, et al. Safety and efficacy of fistula closure by endoscopic suturing: a multi-center study. Endoscopy 2016;48(11):1023–8 [published Online First: 2016/10/28].
58. Jin D, Xu M, Huang K, et al. The efficacy and long-term outcomes of endoscopic full-thickness suturing for chronic gastrointestinal fistulas with an Overstitch device: is it a durable closure? Surg Endosc 2022;36(2):1347–54 [published Online First: 2021/11/19].
59. Susstrunk J, Thumshirn M, Peterli R, et al. Early gastrogastric fistula after Roux-en-Y gastric bypass: successful fistula treatment with self-expandable endoscopic stent. BMJ Case Rep 2021;14(6). https://doi.org/10.1136/bcr-2021-243748 [published Online First: 2021/06/13].

60. Jafri SA, Jay Roberts DO, Smith A. Successful management of early gastrogastric fistula using fully covered esophageal stent. Surg Obes Relat Dis 2018; 14(12):1911–3 [published Online First: 2018/12/14].
61. de Moura DTH, da Ponte-Neto AM, Hathorn KE, et al. Novel Endoscopic Management of a Chronic Gastro-Gastric Fistula Using a Cardiac Septal Defect Occluder. Obes Surg 2020;30(8):3253–4 [published Online First: 2020/04/24].
62. Chahine E, Kassir R, Dirani M, et al. Surgical Management of Gastrogastric Fistula After Roux-en-Y Gastric Bypass: 10-Year Experience. Obes Surg 2018;28(4): 939–44 [published Online First: 2017/10/07].
63. Eisenberg D, Azagury DE, Ghiassi S, et al. ASMBS Position Statement on Postprandial Hyperinsulinemic Hypoglycemia after Bariatric Surgery. Surg Obes Relat Dis 2017;13(3):371–8 [published Online First: 2017/01/24].
64. Vargas EJ, Abu Dayyeh BK, Storm AC, et al. Endoscopic management of dumping syndrome after Roux-en-Y gastric bypass: a large international series and proposed management strategy. Gastrointest Endosc 2020;92(1):91–6 [published Online First: 2020/03/01].
65. Tsai C, Steffen R, Kessler U, et al. Short-term outcomes of endoscopic gastrojejunal revisions for treatment of dumping syndrome after Roux-En-Y gastric bypass. Surg Endosc 2020;34(8):3626–32 [published Online First: 2019/09/26].
66. Bazarbashi AN, Dolan RD, McCarty TR, et al. Endoscopic revision of gastrojejunal anastomosis for the treatment of dumping syndrome in patients with Roux-en-Y gastric bypass: a systematic review and meta-analysis. Surg Endosc 2022; 36(6):4099–107 [published Online First: 2021/10/21].
67. Rebibo L, Hakim S, Dhahri A, et al. Gastric Stenosis After Laparoscopic Sleeve Gastrectomy: Diagnosis and Management. Obes Surg 2016;26(5):995–1001 [published Online First: 2015/09/14].
68. Yu JX, Baker JR, Watts L, et al. Functional Lumen Imaging Probe Is Useful for the Quantification of Gastric Sleeve Stenosis and Prediction of Response to Endoscopic Dilation: a Pilot Study. Obes Surg 2020;30(2):786–9 [published Online First: 2019/07/28].
69. Yu JX, Dolan RD, Bhalla S, et al. Quantification of gastric sleeve stenosis using endoscopic parameters and image analysis. Gastrointest Endosc 2021;93(6): 1344–8 [published Online First: 2020/12/15].
70. Shnell M, Fishman S, Eldar S, et al. Balloon dilatation for symptomatic gastric sleeve stricture. Gastrointest Endosc 2014;79(3):521–4 [published Online First: 2013/11/14].
71. Lorenzo D, Gkolfakis P, Lemmers A, et al. Endoscopic Dilation of Post-Sleeve Gastrectomy Stenosis: Long-Term Efficacy and Safety Results. Obes Surg 2021;31(5):2188–96 [published Online First: 2021/02/19].
72. Donatelli G, Dumont JL, Pourcher G, et al. Pneumatic dilation for functional helix stenosis after sleeve gastrectomy: long-term follow-up (with videos). Surg Obes Relat Dis 2017;13(6):943–50 [published Online First: 2016/12/14].
73. Manos T, Nedelcu M, Cotirlet A, et al. How to treat stenosis after sleeve gastrectomy? Surg Obes Relat Dis 2017;13(2):150–4 [published Online First: 2016/12/21].
74. Agnihotri A, Barola S, Hill C, et al. An Algorithmic Approach to the Management of Gastric Stenosis Following Laparoscopic Sleeve Gastrectomy. Obes Surg 2017; 27(10):2628–36 [published Online First: 2017/05/05].
75. Brunaldi VO, Galvao Neto M, Zundel N, et al. Isolated sleeve gastrectomy stricture: a systematic review on reporting, workup, and treatment. Surg Obes Relat Dis 2020;16(7):955–66 [published Online First: 2020/04/26].

Management of Monogenic and Syndromic Obesity

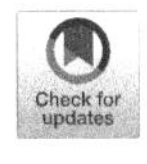

Joan C. Han, MD[a,b,c,*], Marcus C. Rasmussen, BA[a], Alison R. Forte, BA[a], Stephanie B. Schrage, BA[a], Sarah K. Zafar, BA[a], Andrea M. Haqq, MD[d,e]

KEYWORDS

- Leptin • Proopiomelanocortin • Metreleptin • Setmelanotide
- Bardet-Biedl syndrome • Prader-Willi syndrome • Ciliopathy • Syndromic obesity
- Monogenic obesity

KEY POINTS

- Monogenic defects of the leptin pathway cause severe, early childhood-onset obesity.
- Multiple syndromic obesity disorders also converge on the leptin pathway.
- Treatments targeting the leptin pathway provide a precision medicine approach to treating many of these genetic obesity disorders.

INTRODUCTION

The adipocyte-secreted hormone leptin and its downstream signaling mediators within the central nervous system (**Fig. 1**) have been fundamental in understanding energy homeostasis. Targeted pharmacotherapy (**Table 1**) has entered clinical practice for treating obesity associated with monogenetic defects of leptin, leptin receptor (LEPR), POMC, and prohormone convertase 1 and Bardet-Biedl syndrome (BBS), a group of ciliopathies that disrupts several mediators of leptin signaling. A similar precision medicine approach has led to investigational therapies for other leptin pathway defects and syndromic hyperphagic obesity disorders, including Prader-Willi syndrome (PWS).

[a] Division of Pediatric Endocrinology and Diabetes, Department of Pediatrics, Icahn School of Medicine at Mount Sinai, New York, NY, USA; [b] Diabetes, Obesity, and Metabolism Institute, Icahn School of Medicine at Mount Sinai, New York, NY, USA; [c] The Mindich Child Health and Development Institute, Icahn School of Medicine at Mount Sinai, New York, NY, USA; [d] Department of Pediatrics, Faculty of Medicine and Dentistry, University of Alberta, Edmonton, Alberta, Canada; [e] Department of Agricultural, Food and Nutritional Science, University of Alberta, Edmonton, Alberta, Canada
* Corresponding author. Division of Pediatric Endocrinology and Diabetes, Icahn School of Medicine at Mount Sinai, 1468 Madison Avenue, Box 1616, New York, NY 10029.
E-mail address: joan.han@mssm.edu

Gastroenterol Clin N Am 52 (2023) 733–750
https://doi.org/10.1016/j.gtc.2023.08.005
gastro.theclinics.com

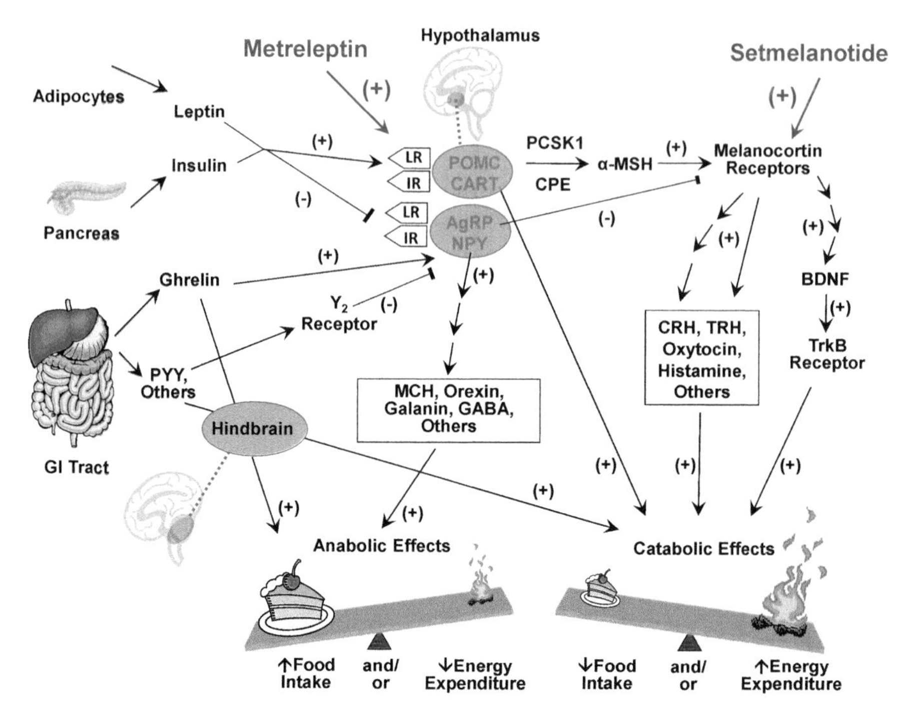

Fig. 1. Targeted sites of therapy within the leptin pathway. In this simplified diagram of the leptin pathway, *lines with arrowheads* show stimulatory action while lines with perpendicular end blocks show inhibitory action. Metreleptin is a ligand for the leptin receptor (LR). Setmelanotide is a ligand for the melanocortin-4 receptor. AgRP, agouti-related protein; BDNF, brain-derived neurotrophic factor; CART, cocaine-amphetamine related transcript; CPE, carboxypeptidase E; CRH, corticotropin-releasing hormone; GABA, gamma amino butyric acid; GI, gastrointestinal; IR, insulin receptor; LR, leptin receptor; MCH, melanin-concentrating hormone; MSH, melanocyte-stimulating hormone; NPY, neuropeptide Y; PCK1, proprotein convertase subtilisin/kexin type 1; POMC, proopiomelanocortin; PYY, peptide YY; TRH, thyrotropin-releasing hormone; TrkB, tropomyosin receptor kinase B. (Reprinted with permission from Elsevier. Han JC et al. The Lancet. 2010 May 15;375(9727):1737-48.)

METRELEPTIN FOR LEPTIN DEFICIENCY

Metreleptin is a recombinant methionyl leptin analog and has a longer half-life than endogenous leptin, permitting once-daily administration. In children with congenital leptin deficiency due to homozygous leptin gene (*LEP*) mutations – leading to undetectable, reduced, or detectable but bioinactive leptin – metreleptin induces significant weight loss due to reduced fat mass while maintaining lean body mass and statural growth.[1–4] Metreleptin also restored the neuroendocrine and immune system abnormalities associated with leptin deficiency, including central hypothyroidism, hypogonadotropic hypogonadism, and defective lymphocyte function.[2,5,6] The development of neutralizing antibodies to metreleptin has been observed, which may pose a challenge for long-term therapy.[2] Currently, the only United States Food and Drug Administration (US-FDA)-approved indication for metreleptin is the treatment of generalized lipodystrophy, which causes hypoleptinemia due to near-total absence or destruction of adipocytes. The metabolic derangements of lipodystrophy mirror those of leptin deficiency, including hyperphagia, steatohepatitis,

Table 1
Targeted pharmacotherapies for monogenic and syndromic causes of obesity converging on the leptin pathway

Monogenetic Disorders	Targeted Pharmacotherapy	Benefits	Challenges	Approved Indications (Obesity-Related)
Leptin Deficiency	Metreleptin *Recombinant methionyl leptin analogue*	Reduction of fat while maintaining lean body mass Restored immune functions associated with leptin deficiency	Development of antibodies to metreleptin may pose a challenge to long-term treatment	Only approved for lipodystrophy, not leptin deficiency or obesity
Leptin Receptor (LEPR) Deficiency Proopiomelanocortin (POMC) Deficiency Proprotein Convertase Subtilisin/Kexin Type 1 (PCSK1) Deficiency	Setmelanotide *MC4R agonist*	Unlike previous MC4R agonists, no significant cardiovascular adverse effects reported Increased resting energy expenditure, appetite suppression	Injection site reactions, skin hyperpigmentation (due to melanocortin-1 receptor activation), nausea, headache, diarrhea, abdominal pain, back pain, fatigue, vomiting, depression, upper respiratory tract infection, and spontaneous penile erection	Obesity in patients aged ≥6 y with LEPR, POMC, or PCSK1 deficiency
Melanocortin-4 Receptor (MC4R) Deficiency	Setmelanotide *MC4R agonist*	Specific variants of MC4R may be rescued	Targeted therapies for MC4R variants unresponsive to this analog are needed	Under investigation

Syndromic Disorders	Targeted Pharmacotherapy	Benefits	Challenges	Approved Indications (Obesity-Related)
Bardet-Biedl syndrome (BBS) Alström syndrome (AS)	Setmelanotide	Above	Above	Approved for BBS but still under investigation for AS

(*continued on next page*)

Table 1
(continued)

Syndromic Disorders	Targeted Pharmacotherapy	Benefits	Challenges	Approved Indications (Obesity-Related)
PWS	Growth hormone therapy	Enhanced growth and motor development, decreased fat mass and increased lean mass, improved energy expenditure May improve neurodevelopment if begun in infancy	No significant adverse effects, but monitoring of glucose metabolism, cardiovascular disease, sleep-disordered breathing, scoliosis, and longer-term cancer risk is advised	PWS
	Liraglutide and Semaglutide *Glucagon-like peptide-1 receptor agonists*	Appetite suppression and delayed gastric emptying	Gastrointestinal disorders	Obesity in patients ≥12 y of age
	Oxytocin and Carbetocin *Neuropeptide and its synthetic analogue* PWS	May reduce appetite and social function deficits	Symptoms of anxiety, facial flushing	Under investigation
	Ghrelin modulators *Analog of unacylated ghrelin* *Inhibition of ghrelin-O-acyltransferase*	May improve hyperphagia and post-prandial glucose concentration	No significant adverse effects reported	Under investigation
	Diazoxide choline *Benzothiadiazine that acts through ATP-sensitive K+ channels*	May reduce appetite and decrease fat mass	Hypertrichosis, peripheral edema, and hyperglycemia	Under investigation
	Belanorib *Methionine aminopeptidase-2 inhibitor*	May reduce appetite and decrease fat mass	Injection site bruising, venous thrombotic events	Analogs that do not cause increased thrombosis are under investigation
	Combination of tesofensine and metoprolol *Monoamine reuptake inhibitors + beta-1 selective blocker*	May reduce appetite and body weight	Sleep disturbances, dry mouth, headache, and exacerbation of pre-existing anxiety	Under investigation with FDA Orphan Drug Designation for PWS and hypothalamic obesity

hypertriglyceridemia, severe insulin resistance, and type 2 diabetes which are all ameliorated by metreleptin therapy.[7,8]

SETMELANOTIDE FOR LEPR, POMC, AND PCSK1 DEFICIENCIES

Binding of leptin to the LEPR leads activation of neurons that express POMC, a peptide prohormone that is cleaved by PCSK1 to produce α-melanocyte-stimulating hormone (α-MSH), the endogenous ligand of the melanocortin-4 receptor (MC4R), and several other peptides, and adrenocorticotrophic hormone (ACTH). Biallelic deleterious mutations of the genes encoding LEPR, POMC, and PCSK1 cause rare autosomal recessive monogenic obesity, characterized by severe hyperphagia and development of obesity in early childhood. Clinically, LEPR deficiency is similar in phenotype to leptin deficiency.[9,10] POMC deficiency is associated with adrenal insufficiency due to ACTH deficiency and hypopigmentation because of melanin induced by α-MSH activation of the melanocortin-1 receptor (MC1R) in skin and hair.[11] PCSK1 deficiency causes reduced processing of several other prohormone peptides besides POMC, including proglucagon and proinsulin, conferring additional features, including malabsorptive diarrhea and post-prandial hyperglycemia due to insulin insufficiency, followed by hypoglycemia mediated by elevated residual proinsulin.[12,13]

Unlike earlier MC4R agonists which induced hypertension and tachycardia as untoward side effects,[14] setmelanotide is an MC1R and MC4R agonist that avoids appreciable sympathetic nervous system activation in primates, making it an attractive therapeutic for bypassing the deficits caused by LEPR, POMC, and PCSK1 deficiencies.[15,16] In adults with obesity and no known genetic abnormalities, short-term 72-h setmelanotide administration increased resting-energy expenditure without adverse cardiovascular effects.[17] In a 4-week randomized-controlled trial (RCT), setmelanotide induced a modest 4% (placebo-subtracted) reduction in weight.[16] Studies of setmelanotide soon followed in patients with genetic conditions affecting the leptin-melanocortin pathway. In open-label trials of patients aged ≥6 years with LEPR, POMC, or PCSK1 deficiency, setmelanotide significantly reduced hunger and induced at least 10% weight loss at ~12 months in 45% of patients with LEPR deficiency, 80% of patients with POMC deficiency, and 80% of patients with PCSK1 deficiency.[18,19] Common adverse events included injection-site reactions, skin hyperpigmentation (due to MC1R activation), nausea, headache, diarrhea, abdominal pain, back pain, fatigue, vomiting, depression, upper-respiratory-tract infection, and spontaneous penile erection.[20] Setmelanotide received US-FDA approval in November 2020 for treatment of obesity in patients aged ≥6 years with LEPR, POMC, or PCSK1 deficiency. The efficacy of setmelanotide for treatment of obesity associated with deficiency of carboxypeptidase E, an additional processing enzyme for PCSK1, is currently under investigation (ClinicalTrials.gov Identifier: NCT04963231).[21]

MC4R DEFICIENCY

Mutations of MC4R that impair its synthesis, plasma membrane expression, ligand binding capacity, intracellular signaling, or recycling after endocytosis can cause obesity in an autosomal dominant pattern of inheritance.[22] Homozygous and compound heterozygous (ie, biallelic) *MC4R* mutations are rare and cause extreme obesity, while heterozygous mutations cause less severe obesity and are fairly common, reported in approximately 3% of patients with childhood-onset obesity.[23,24] Interventions used in common forms of obesity, such as liraglutide, phentermine, and bariatric surgery, may have some short-term efficacy in individuals with MC4R mutations, but a frequent observation is attenuated responsiveness and weight regain, particularly for patients with biallelic MC4R mutations.[25–29] Targeted therapies are therefore needed. Setmelanotide did not induce statistically significant weight loss in a small cohort of adults with a variety of heterozygous MC4R mutations, but whether genotype-specific responsiveness in vitro for the greater-than-350 MC4R known variants can predict responsiveness in vivo remains to be explored.[16] Novel investigations include translational readthrough enhancers to overcome stop codons, chaperones to enhance misfolded receptor trafficking, modifiers of dimerization, and targeting of downstream signaling mediators.[30,31]

CILIOPATHIES CONVERGING ON THE LEPTIN PATHWAY

BBS and Alström syndrome (AS) are rare, autosomal recessive ciliopathies caused by mutations in one of greater-than-20 BBS genes (*BBS1-BBS22*) or the *ALMS1* gene. Patients develop early childhood-onset hyperphagia[32] and obesity plus retinal dystrophy, renal disease, and gonadal dysfunction.[33,34] Patients with BBS also typically have polydactyly and intellectual deficiency,[33] while AS is often associated with hearing loss and cardiomyopathy but preserved cognitive function.[34,35] The mechanism for the appetite dysregulation and weight gain in both BBS and AS is attributed to leptin resistance[36,37] due to the role of cilia in LEPR transport to the plasma membrane and POMC neuronal survival and function.[38–40] Bypassing the defects in LEPR and POMC of patients with ciliopathy disorders by activation of MC4R with setmelanotide has been demonstrated to be an effective approach. In an open-label study of patients with BBS aged ≥12 years, setmelanotide treatment for 52 weeks resulted in 16.3% weight loss after 52 weeks.[41] In a subsequent RCT, 32.3% of patients with BBS had at least a 10% reduction in body weight after 52 weeks of setmelanotide with a mean reduction in weight by 9.5%.[42] Setmelanotide received FDA approval for the treatment of obesity in patients with BBS in June 2022.

Investigations of setmelanotide in AS have been hampered by low enrollment due the rarity of the condition,[43] but preliminary data of combined 8 patients with AS enrolled in phase 2 and 3 studies (ClinicalTrials.gov Identifiers: NCT03013543, NCT03746522) showed that in patients who received setmelanotide for 9.7 to 18.2 months, 1 of 2 adults (50%) had ≥25% decrease in hunger score; 5 of 6 (83.3%) youth younger than 18 years achieved ≥0.2 decrease in body mass index (BMI) Z-score; 3 of 4 patients (75%) aged ≥12 to less than 18 years achieved ≥25% hunger score decrease; 2 of 8 patients (25%) had improved QOL. Overall, 7 of 8 patients (87.5%) had improvement in at least one of the outcome domains. These findings are encouraging and warrant further studies of setmelanotide in AS, in particular, the role of patient genotype or other characteristics as predictors of response.[44]

Specific dietary recommendations may also benefit BBS and AS because both are associated with insulin resistance that is more severe than expected for degree of adiposity,[36,37] which may be attributable to the role of primary cilia in insulin receptor signaling.[45] Therefore, caloric portion control, physical activity, and limiting of simple carbohydrate intake are recommended in patients with ciliopathy-associated obesity.[35,46] Data regarding the safety and efficacy of bariatric surgery in such patients are limited, with a few case reports showing moderate weight loss but of uncertain sustainability[29] and lack of impact on type 2 diabetes control in the case of gastric banding.[47,48]

TREATMENT OF PRADER-WILLI SYNDROME

PWS is caused by a lack of expression of paternal genes located in the chromosome 15q11.2-q13 region caused by paternal gene deletion (70%), maternal uniparental disomy (25%), or imprinting defects (5%).[49] PWS is characterized by poor feeding during

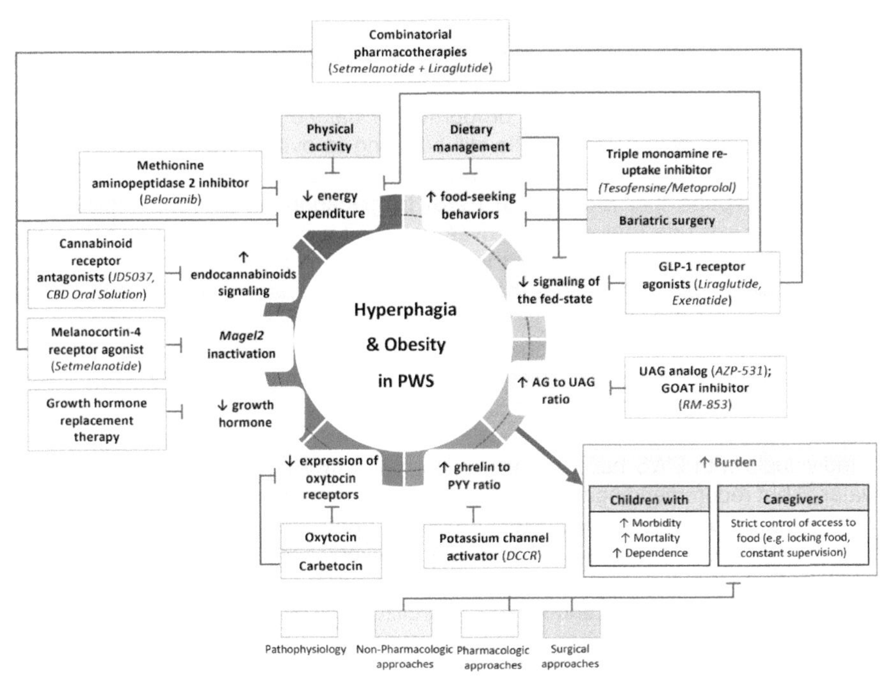

Fig. 2. Pathophysiology of Prader-Willi syndrome and treatment approaches. Emerging therapies under investigation for the treatment of hyperphagia and obesity in Prader-Willi syndrome include pharmacologic (medication names shown in italics), nonpharmacologic, and surgical approaches to target specific mechanistic aspects of the syndrome. AG, acylated ghrelin; AG, unacylated ghrelin; DCCR, diazoxide choline controlled release; GLP-1, glucagon-like peptide 1; GOAT, ghrelin O-acyltransferase; PYY, peptide YY. (*From* Tan, Q, Orsso, CE, Deehan, EC, et al. Current and emerging therapies for managing hyperphagia and obesity in Prader-Willi syndrome: A narrative review. Obesity Reviews. 2020; 21:e12992. https://doi.org/10.1111/obr.12992.)

infancy, followed by progressive weight gain, lack of satiety, and constant food-seeking behaviors. A framework for PWS management is shown in **Fig. 2**.

Nutrition Recommendations in Prader-Willi Syndrome

Involvement of parents and all caregivers is necessary to have control of the environment with regard to food access and consistent scheduling of meals and snacks consumption and physical activity.[50] Restriction of food access is necessary to prevent hyperphagic overeating, which can become so severe if unmonitored as to cause gastric necrosis.[51] Establishing a routine for timing of food intake is beneficial for reducing anxiety about food access and preventing behavior problems, such as temper tantrums, manipulation, and sneaking.[52]

Energy needs are less in individuals with PWS due to lower lean muscle mass and higher percentage body fat than age-, sex-, and BMI-matched controls.[53,54] Therefore, dietary recommendations for infants and children with PWS are approximately 20% to 40% fewer calories to maintain energy balance than for healthy individuals of the same age.[53,55] For weight maintenance, 10.0 to 14.0 kcal/cm of height is recommended, and for weight reduction, 7 to 9 kcal/cm of height.[56,57] Close monitoring is necessary to prevent overrestriction, which could worsen hunger drive and behavioral exacerbations and cause micronutrient deficiencies.[58] Lower carbohydrate consumption and higher dietary fiber intake (at least 20 g/day) have been generally recommended for patients with PWS,[59] but even stricter limitation of carbohydrates in favor of increased proportion of calories from fats (15% carbohydrates; 65% fat; 20% protein) while still adhering to overall energy-reduced intake has been proposed as a beneficial approach for reducing the ratio of ghrelin (an orexigenic peptide that is higher in PWS) to glucagon-like peptide 1 (GLP-1, an anorexigenic peptide that also improves beta-cell function and insulin sensitivity), thereby reducing hunger drive and improving glycemic control.[60] Increasing fiber intake even further to 40 g/day has been proposed based on the premise that fermentation of dietary fiber by gut bacteria produces short-chain fatty acids, which promote expression and secretion of GLP-1 and another anorexigenic intestinal hormone, peptide YY.[61] Thus, modulation of the gut by dietary fiber could be a potential treatment strategy in PWS and is currently under investigation (ClinicalTrials.gov Identifier: NCT04150991).

Individuals with PWS have a tendency to prefer sweetened beverages over plain water,[62] but recommending the use of nonnutritive sweeteners should be approached with caution and avoided if possible due to the potential negative impact on the intestinal microbiome and the hedonic response to sweetness, which could worsen hunger.[63,64] Probiotic supplementation has been proposed, but studies are limited to short-term trials. A 4-week randomized controlled crossover study examining probiotics for treatment of constipation in PWS showed minimal effect on laxation and microbiota composition.[65] A 12-week RCT in 71 individuals with PWS resulted in BMI reduction and improvements in neurodevelopmental measures within the probiotic group.[66] Further studies are needed to assess optimal diet composition for weight management in PWS.

Growth hormone therapy in Prader-Willi syndrome

Short stature and growth hormone (GH) deficiency are common patients with PWS.[67] GH therapy, approved for growth promotion in children with PWS by the US-FDA and Health Canada, has positive benefits during childhood on height, motor development, body composition (decreased fat mass and increased lean mass), and energy expenditure,[68] plus potential benefits for neurodevelopment when begun in infancy in some studies.[69] In adults with PWS, GH treatment has continued benefits on body composition, muscle strength, exercise capacity, and quality of life.[70,71] Current standards of care in PWS support the early use of GH therapy as soon as possible after genetic confirmation of PWS diagnosis.[72,73] Treatment has generally been safe with no significant adverse effects on glucose metabolism, cardiovascular disease, sleep-disordered breathing, scoliosis, or longer-term cancer risk, although close monitoring for these complications is still advised.[74]

Glucagon-like peptide-1 receptor agonists in Prader-Willi syndrome

GLP-1 receptor agonists (GLP1RAs) induce weight loss via appetite suppression and delayed gastric emptying. A systematic review of 10 studies summarizing nonrandomized exenatide or liraglutide use in 23 patients with PWS (aged 13–37 years) over 14 weeks to 4 years reported improvements in BMI (1.5–16 kg/m^2), hemoglobin A1C in 19 of 23 cases, and satiety.[75] A recently published RCT including 55 children and adolescents with PWS who received 3 mg (or maximum tolerated dose) liraglutide or placebo (randomized 2:1) for 16 weeks followed by liraglutide for 52 weeks while participating in a structured diet and exercise program.[76] There were no significant differences between groups for change in BMI SDS (for age and sex standards) at 16 or

52 weeks, although hyperphagia was lower in adolescents treated with liraglutide than placebo at 52 weeks.[76] The most common adverse events with liraglutide were gastrointestinal disorders.[76] RCTs of more potent GLP1RAs, such as semaglutide, or combination therapies such as glucose-dependent insulinotropic polypeptide (GIP)/GLP-1 receptor dual agonists (eg, tirzepatide) or GLP-1/GIP/glucagon receptor triagonists (eg, SAR441255)[77] have yet to be explored in PWS. In a case series of 2 patients with PWS who received semaglutide, BMI SDS increased in one and decreased in the other.[78]

Melanocortin-4 receptor agonist in Prader-Willi syndrome

Magel2 is a gene within the PWS chromosome 15 critical region.[49] Magel2-deficient mice have a POMC deficit responsive to pharmacologic treatment with the MC4R agonist setmelanotide.[79] Setmelanotide is currently being investigated as a treatment for hyperphagia and obesity in patients with PWS (ClinicalTrials.gov Identifier: NCT02311673).

Oxytocin and carbetocin in Prader-Willi syndrome

Oxytocin is a neuropeptide that plays a key role in human social behaviors, including parental bonding, trust, and regulation of feeding.[80] Reduced hypothalamic oxytocin-expressing neurons has been observed in PWS,[81] suggesting a potential role in the hyperphagia, anxiety, and social deficits of PWS.[82] Intranasal administration of oxytocin in patients with PWS has been reported as well tolerated and safe, but effects on hyperphagia and social function have been mixed, with possible differences in response based on sex and PWS subtype.[83–88]

Carbetocin is a synthetic analog of oxytocin that is more selective for the oxytocin receptor, which may confer benefits over oxytocin as oxytocin's partial agonism at the arginine vasopressin receptor could contribute to anxiogenic side effects of oxytocin.[85] The results of the largest RCT to date of intranasal carbetocin in 119 patients with PWS (aged 7–18 years) reported that the 8-week placebo-controlled period of the study (carbetocin 9.6 mg, carbetocin 3.2 mg, or matching placebo by nasal spray TID with meals) showed no difference in weight changes between groups; the carbetocin 3.2-mg group (though not the higher 9.6 mg arm) demonstrated significant improvements in hyperphagia, Clinical Global Impression, and PWS Anxiety and Distress Questionnaire, with benefits sustained in the 56-week follow-up period of open-label carbetocin treatment.[89] Intranasal carbetocin was well-tolerated, with flushing as the most frequent adverse event reported.[89]

Ghrelin modulation in Prader-Willi syndrome

Elevation of the active acylated form of the orexigen ghrelin has been observed in PWS,[90] leading to the hypothesis that competitive inhibition using an analog of unacylated ghrelin could oppose the appetite-increasing effect of endogenous acylated ghrelin. Livoletide (AZP-531), a cyclic 8 amino acid analog of unacylated ghrelin A, was observed in a 14-day RCT of 47 patients with PWS (aged 12–50 years) to improve hyperphagia and post-prandial glucose concentration compared to placebo.[91] Livoletide was well-tolerated with no serious side effects. A lack of effect on hyperphagia and body weight of livoletide in a subsequent 12-week RCT led to discontinuation of further studies for this medication.[92]

Inhibition of ghrelin-O-acyltransferase, the enzyme which catalyzes ghrelin acylation, has been studied using GLWL-01 administered at 450 mg po BID in a 28-day double-blind, placebo-controlled phase 2 crossover study in 19 patients with PWS.[93] GLWL-01 treatment resulted in a significant reduction in acylated ghrelin, but hyperphagia, eating behaviors, BMI, and metabolic parameters were unchanged. Further longer-term studies are required.

Diazoxide in Prader-Willi syndrome

Diazoxide choline is a benzothiadiazine that acts through ATP-sensitive K+ channels (KATP) and is used for treatment of hyperinsulinemic hypoglycemia. It may exert therapeutic effects in PWS through downregulation of insulin from pancreatic β-cells, decrease in hypothalamic neuropeptide Y concentrations, increase in GABAergic neurons, and/or activation of KATP channels in adipocytes.[94] Diazoxide choline-controlled release (DCCR) is an extended-release form of diazoxide choline. In a 13-week randomized, double-blind, placebo-controlled phase 3 trial, DCCR significantly reduced fat mass ($P = .003$) but without significant difference in BMI.[95] Hyperphagia improved only in patients with severe hyperphagia at baseline.[95] The most common DCCR-associated side effects were hypertrichosis, peripheral edema, and hyperglycemia.[95] Long-term studies are needed.

Methionine aminopeptidase-2 inhibitor (belanorib) in Prader-Willi syndrome

Belanorib is an irreversible inhibitor of methionine aminopeptidase-2 (MetAP2), an enzyme that is implicated in cell growth and angiogenesis. Inhibition of MetAP2 leads to weight loss through several proposed mechanisms, including decreased caloric intake,[96] increased fat mobilization and oxidation, suppression of endothelial cell proliferation,[97] and prevention of adipose tissue expansion.[98] A 26-week phase 3 randomized, double-blind, placebo-controlled trial was conducted of belanorib in 107 participants with PWS (aged 12–65 years).[99] Patients were randomly assigned (1:1:1) to biweekly placebo (n = 34), 1.8 mg of belanorib (n = 36), or 2.4 mg of belanorib (n = 37). Improvement in hyperphagia was seen in the 1.8- and 2.4-mg belanorib groups ($P = .0003$ and $P = .0001$ vs placebo). In addition, weight loss was greater with 1.8 mg or 2.4 mg of belanorib ($P < .0001$ vs placebo). Injection-site bruising was the most common adverse event. However, the trial was terminated early due to venous thrombotic events in the belanorib-treated participants (two with fatal pulmonary embolism). Next-generation MetAP2 inhibitors are under investigation with efficacy for weight loss but with better safety profiles as the goal.

Combination tesofensine and metoprolol in Prader-Willi syndrome

The FDA granted orphan drug designation for fixed-dose combination of tesofensine and metoprolol in PWS in March 2021 and hypothalamic obesity in July 2021. Tesofensine is a centrally acting monoamine reuptake inhibitor that blocks the presynaptic reuptake of dopamine, serotonin, and noradrenaline. Metoprolol is a beta-1 selective blocker dosed at a ratio of 100:1 in combination with tesofensine to prevent adverse cardiovascular effects (tachycardia and hypertension) commonly associated with tesofensine and other monoamine reuptake inhibitors, such as sibutramine. In unpublished data (https://www.globenewswire.com/news-release/2021/03/03/2186073/0/en/Saniona-Receives-U-S-FDA-Orphan-Drug-Designation-for-Tesomet-in-Prader-Willi-Syndrome.html) supplied by the manufacturer from a randomized, double-blind, placebo-controlled phase 2a trial (ClinicalTrials.gov Identifier: NCT03149445), adults with PWS receiving tesofensine/metoprolol had a statistically significant reduction in hyperphagia and a clinically meaningful reduction in body weight at a dose of 0.5 mg of tesofensine/50 mg of metoprolol daily while adolescents with PWS had positive responses at lower doses.[100] The only published data on tesofensine/metoprolol are from a study of 21 adults with hypothalamic obesity randomized to receive 0.5 mg of tesofensine/50 mg of metoprolol or placebo for 24 weeks.[101] Adverse events associated with tesofensine/metoprolol included sleep disturbances, dry mouth, headache, and exacerbation of pre-existing anxiety. There were no significant differences in heart rate or blood pressure between treatment groups. The difference between tesofensine/metoprolol and placebo was a mean weight change of −6.3% (95% CI: −11.3, −1.3; $P = .017$). A phase 2b clinical trial in patients with PWS (ClinicalTrials.gov Identifier: NCT05198362) was initiated in December 2021 but voluntarily suspended by the manufacturer in March 2022 due to financial constraints.

OTHER ANTI-OBESITY MEDICATIONS IN PRADER-WILLI SYNDROME

Currently available FDA-approved long-term medications for obesity treatment in the general population include orlistat, GLP1RAs (liraglutide, semaglutide), and phentermine/topiramate for patients aged ≥12 years and bupropion/naltrexone in adults. Data for orlistat in PWS are lacking in the extant literature. GLP1RAs in PWS are discussed previously. Data for phentermine/topiramate and bupropion/naltrexone in PWS are limited to case series reports,[101,102] but overall, these medications appear to show efficacy and safety profiles in PWS similar to the general population although discontinuation rates were high, particularly for phentermine/topiramate due to side effects, and weight regain occurred with discontinuation. The endocannabinoid receptor CB1 antagonist, rimonabant, which had been initially approved for the treatment of obesity in Europe in 2006, was postulated to be particularly beneficial in individuals with PWS too because of the increased endocannabinoid tone that has been observed in PWS.[103] However, the severe adverse psychiatric effects observed in the general population, as well as in patients with PWS,[104] led to withdrawal of rimonabant from clinical use in 2008. Peripherally restricted endocannabinoid receptor CB1 antagonists have been proposed as a potential alternative approach that may avoid these side effects, but no data from clinical trials have been reported to date.[103]

Bariatric Surgery in Prader-Willi Syndrome

A recent systematic review of metabolic and bariatric surgery (MBS) in PWS (67 patients from 22 articles evaluated outcomes of laparoscopic sleeve gastrectomy (LSG), gastric bypass (GB), and biliopancreatic diversion (BPD). No mortality within 1 year was reported in any of the 3 groups after a primary MBS operation. All groups experienced a significant decrease in BMI at 1 year with a mean reduction in BMI of 14.7 kg/m^2 ($P < .001$) with sustained weight loss in the LSG, GB, and BPD groups for up to 3, 2, and 7 years, respectively.[105] Iron deficiency was reported for 1 patient in the LSG group and 1 patient in the BPD group; 2 cases of osteoporosis were reported in the BPD group.[105] No nutritional deficiencies were reported in the GB group.[105] Additional long-term studies are needed for the safety and efficacy of bariatric surgery in PWS.

CONCLUSIONS AND FUTURE DIRECTIONS

Bypassing defects within the leptin signaling pathway is an effective approach for obesity treatment in specific disorders: metreleptin for leptin deficiency and setmelanotide for defects of the LEPR, POMC, and its processor, PCSK1, as well as ciliopathies that affect the leptin pathway. Whether this approach may be beneficial for treating obesity in heterozygous carriers of common variants in these same genes is under investigation (ClinicalTrials.gov Identifier: NCT05093634). Furthermore, emerging combination of anti-obesity drugs such as tirzepatide (GIP/GLP1RAs) or retatrutide (GIP/GLP-1/glucagon receptor triagonist) warrant further study in genetic obesity conditions. Finally, novel approaches of targeting downstream mediators of the leptin pathway, such as brain-derived neurotrophic factor (BDNF), show promise. In a Magel2-null mouse model for PWS, adeno-associate virusmediated hypothalamic gene transfer of BDNF decreased fat mass without inducing cachexia due to an autoregulatory mechanism in which silencing RNA for BDNF is produced under the control of an agouti-related protein (AgRP) responsive promoter that is activated by the increase in AgRP secretion that occurs in the setting of excessive weight loss.[106] Augmenting BDNF and other downstream mediators of the leptin pathway hold potential for the treatment of other genetic causes of obesity beyond PWS as there are dozens of other syndromic conditions associated with obesity for which such an approach could be beneficial.[107]

CLINICS CARE POINTS

- Metreleptin, a leptin analogue with a longer half-life, reduces adiposity in patients with leptin deficiency, but the development of neutralizing antibodies may diminish efficacy.
- Setmelanotide, a melanocortin-4 receptor agonist, is FDA-approved for the treatment of obesity in patients aged ≥6 years with LEPR, POMC, or PCSK1 deficiency or who have Bardet-Biedl syndrome.
- In patients with Prader-Willi syndrome, growth hormone increases lean mass and reduces adiposity. Liraglutide and semaglutide, glucagon-like peptide-1 receptor agonists, reduce appetite, but their effect on BMI in PWS is equivocal. Multiple studies of investigational therapies for PWS are currently ongoing.

DISCLOSURE

J.C. Han is a clinical trial investigator for multi-site research studies sponsored by Rhythm Pharmaceuticals. A.M. Haqq is a clinical trial investigator for multi-site research studies sponsored by Rhythm Pharmaceuticals, Levo Therapeutics, and Eli Lilly. She has received grants from the Weston Family Microbiome Initiative and Canadian Institutes of Health Research, Canada, payment as a speaker for Pfizer Canada, and is a member of advisory boards for Pfizer, Rhythm Pharmaceuticals, and Novo Nordisk Canada. The remaining authors have no disclosures.

REFERENCES

1. Montague CT, Farooqi IS, Whitehead JP, et al. Congenital leptin deficiency is associated with severe early-onset obesity in humans. Nature 1997;387(6636):903–8.
2. Farooqi IS, Matarese G, Lord GM, et al. Beneficial effects of leptin on obesity, T cell hyporesponsiveness, and neuroendocrine/metabolic dysfunction of human congenital leptin deficiency. J Clin Invest 2002;110(8):1093–103.
3. Wabitsch M, Funcke JB, von Schnurbein J, et al. Severe Early-Onset Obesity Due to Bioinactive Leptin Caused by a p.N103K Mutation in the Leptin Gene. J Clin Endocrinol Metab 2015;100(9):3227–30.
4. Wabitsch M, Pridzun L, Ranke M, et al. Measurement of immunofunctional leptin to detect and monitor patients with functional leptin deficiency. Eur J Endocrinol 2017;176(3):315–22.
5. Mantzoros CS, Flier JS, Rogol AD. A longitudinal assessment of hormonal and physical alterations during normal puberty in boys. V. Rising leptin levels may signal the onset of puberty. J Clin Endocrinol Metab 1997;82(4):1066–70.
6. Mantzoros CS, Ozata M, Negrao AB, et al. Synchronicity of frequently sampled thyrotropin (TSH) and leptin concentrations in healthy adults and leptin-deficient

subjects: evidence for possible partial TSH regulation by leptin in humans. J Clin Endocrinol Metab 2001;86(7):3284–91.
7. Javor ED, Cochran EK, Musso C, et al. Long-term efficacy of leptin replacement in patients with generalized lipodystrophy. Diabetes 2005;54(7):1994–2002.
8. Oral EA, Simha V, Ruiz E, et al. Leptin-replacement therapy for lipodystrophy. N Engl J Med 2002;346(8):570–8.
9. Clement K, Vaisse C, Lahlou N, et al. A mutation in the human leptin receptor gene causes obesity and pituitary dysfunction. Nature 1998;392(6674):398–401.
10. Farooqi IS, Wangensteen T, Collins S, et al. Clinical and molecular genetic spectrum of congenital deficiency of the leptin receptor. N Engl J Med 2007;356(3): 237–47.
11. Krude H, Biebermann H, Luck W, et al. Severe early-onset obesity, adrenal insufficiency and red hair pigmentation caused by POMC mutations in humans. Nat Genet 1998;19(2):155–7.
12. Frank GR, Fox J, Candela N, et al. Severe obesity and diabetes insipidus in a patient with PCSK1 deficiency. Mol Genet Metab 2013;110(1–2):191–4.
13. O'Rahilly S, Gray H, Humphreys PJ, et al. Brief report: impaired processing of prohormones associated with abnormalities of glucose homeostasis and adrenal function. N Engl J Med 1995;333(21):1386–90.
14. Greenfield JR, Miller JW, Keogh JM, et al. Modulation of blood pressure by central melanocortinergic pathways. N Engl J Med 2009;360(1):44–52.
15. Kievit P, Halem H, Marks DL, et al. Chronic treatment with a melanocortin-4 receptor agonist causes weight loss, reduces insulin resistance, and improves cardiovascular function in diet-induced obese rhesus macaques. Diabetes 2013;62(2):490–7.
16. Collet TH, Dubern B, Mokrosinski J, et al. Evaluation of a melanocortin-4 receptor (MC4R) agonist (Setmelanotide) in MC4R deficiency. Mol Metab 2017;6(10): 1321–9.
17. Chen KY, Muniyappa R, Abel BS, et al. RM-493, a melanocortin-4 receptor (MC4R) agonist, increases resting energy expenditure in obese individuals. J Clin Endocrinol Metab 2015;100(4):1639–45.
18. Clement K, van den Akker E, Argente J, et al. Efficacy and safety of setmelanotide, an MC4R agonist, in individuals with severe obesity due to LEPR or POMC deficiency: single-arm, open-label, multicentre, phase 3 trials. Lancet Diabetes Endocrinol 2020;8(12):960–70.
19. Wabitsch M, Farooqi S, Fluck CE, et al. Natural History of Obesity Due to POMC, PCSK1, and LEPR Deficiency and the Impact of Setmelanotide. J Endocr Soc 2022;6(6):bvac057.
20. Kanti V, Puder L, Jahnke I, et al. A Melanocortin-4 Receptor Agonist Induces Skin and Hair Pigmentation in Patients with Monogenic Mutations in the Leptin-Melanocortin Pathway. Skin Pharmacol Physiol 2021;34(6):307–16.
21. Alsters SI, Goldstone AP, Buxton JL, et al. Truncating Homozygous Mutation of Carboxypeptidase E (CPE) in a Morbidly Obese Female with Type 2 Diabetes Mellitus, Intellectual Disability and Hypogonadotrophic Hypogonadism. PLoS One 2015;10(6):e0131417.
22. Tao YX. Mutations in melanocortin-4 receptor: From fish to men. Prog Mol Biol Transl Sci 2022;189(1):215–57.
23. Farooqi IS, Keogh JM, Yeo GS, et al. Clinical spectrum of obesity and mutations in the melanocortin 4 receptor gene. N Engl J Med 2003;348(12):1085–95.

24. Drabkin M, Birk OS, Birk R. Heterozygous versus homozygous phenotype caused by the same MC4R mutation: novel mutation affecting a large consanguineous kindred. BMC Med Genet 2018;19(1):135.
25. Salazar-Valencia IG, Villamil-Ramirez H, Barajas-Olmos F, et al. Effect of the Melanocortin 4-Receptor Ile269Asn Mutation on Weight Loss Response to Dietary, Phentermine and Bariatric Surgery Interventions. Genes 2022;13(12). https://doi.org/10.3390/genes13122267.
26. Grinbaum R, Beglaibter N, Mitrani-Rosenbaum S, et al. The Obesogenic and Glycemic Effect of Bariatric Surgery in a Family with a Melanocortin 4 Receptor Loss-of-Function Mutation. Metabolites 2022;12(5). https://doi.org/10.3390/metabo12050430.
27. Cooiman MI, Alsters SIM, Duquesnoy M, et al. Long-Term Weight Outcome After Bariatric Surgery in Patients with Melanocortin-4 Receptor Gene Variants: a Case-Control Study of 105 Patients. Obes Surg 2022;32(3):837–44.
28. Fojas EGF, Radha SK, Ali T, et al. Weight and Glycemic Control Outcomes of Bariatric Surgery and Pharmacotherapy in Patients With Melanocortin-4 Receptor Deficiency. Front Endocrinol 2021;12:792354.
29. Gantz MG, Driscoll DJ, Miller JL, et al. Critical review of bariatric surgical outcomes in patients with Prader-Willi syndrome and other hyperphagic disorders. Obesity 2022;30(5):973–81.
30. Brouwers B, de Oliveira EM, Marti-Solano M, et al. Human MC4R variants affect endocytosis, trafficking and dimerization revealing multiple cellular mechanisms involved in weight regulation. Cell Rep 2021;34(12):108862.
31. Hopfner F, Paisdzior S, Reininghaus N, et al. Evaluation of Pharmacological Rescue of Melanocortin-4 Receptor Nonsense Mutations by Aminoglycoside. Life 2022;12(11). https://doi.org/10.3390/life12111793.
32. Sherafat-Kazemzadeh R, Ivey L, Kahn SR, et al. Hyperphagia among patients with Bardet-Biedl syndrome. Pediatr Obes 2013;8(5):e64–7.
33. Tobin JL, Beales PL. Bardet-Biedl syndrome: beyond the cilium. Pediatr Nephrol 2007;22(7):926–36.
34. Marshall JD, Beck S, Maffei P, et al. Alstrom syndrome. Eur J Hum Genet 2007; 15(12):1193–202.
35. Tahani N, Maffei P, Dollfus H, et al. Consensus clinical management guidelines for Alstrom syndrome. Orphanet J Rare Dis 2020;15(1):253.
36. Feuillan PP, Ng D, Han JC, et al. Patients with Bardet-Biedl syndrome have hyperleptinemia suggestive of leptin resistance. J Clin Endocrinol Metab 2011; 96(3):E528–35.
37. Han JC, Reyes-Capo DP, Liu CY, et al. Comprehensive Endocrine-Metabolic Evaluation of Patients With Alstrom Syndrome Compared With BMI-Matched Controls. J Clin Endocrinol Metab 2018;103(7):2707–19.
38. Guo DF, Cui H, Zhang Q, et al. The BBSome Controls Energy Homeostasis by Mediating the Transport of the Leptin Receptor to the Plasma Membrane. PLoS Genet 2016;12(2):e1005890.
39. Heydet D, Chen LX, Larter CZ, et al. A truncating mutation of Alms1 reduces the number of hypothalamic neuronal cilia in obese mice. Dev Neurobiol 2013; 73(1):1–13.
40. Mariman EC, Vink RG, Roumans NJ, et al. The cilium: a cellular antenna with an influence on obesity risk. Br J Nutr 2016;116(4):576–92.
41. Haws R, Brady S, Davis E, et al. Effect of setmelanotide, a melanocortin-4 receptor agonist, on obesity in Bardet-Biedl syndrome. Diabetes Obes Metab 2020;22(11):2133–40.

42. Haqq AM, Chung WK, Dollfus H, et al. Efficacy and safety of setmelanotide, a melanocortin-4 receptor agonist, in patients with Bardet-Biedl syndrome and Alstrom syndrome: a multicentre, randomised, double-blind, placebo-controlled, phase 3 trial with an open-label period. Lancet Diabetes Endocrinol 2022; 10(12):859–68.
43. Haws RM, Gordon G, Han JC, et al. The efficacy and safety of setmelanotide in individuals with Bardet-Biedl syndrome or Alstrom syndrome: Phase 3 trial design. Contemp Clin Trials Commun 2021;22:100780.
44. Haqq AM, Chung W, Hu S, et al. Clinical Benefit of Setmelanotide in Patients With Alström Syndrome. Abstracts from the 40th Annual Meeting of the Obesity Society (Poster 218). presented at: ObesityWeek; November 1–4, 2022 2022; San Diego, CA.
45. Wang L, Liu Y, Stratigopoulos G, et al. Bardet-Biedl syndrome proteins regulate intracellular signaling and neuronal function in patient-specific iPSC-derived neurons. J Clin Invest 2021;131(8). https://doi.org/10.1172/JCI146287.
46. Paisey RB, Steeds R, Barrett T, et al. Alström Syndrome, In: Adam MP, Ardinger HH and Pagon RA. *GeneReviews® [Internet]*, 2019 (last updated), University of Washington, Seattle; 2003 (initial posting). Available at: https://www.ncbi.nlm.nih.gov/books/NBK1267/.
47. Daskalakis M, Till H, Kiess W, et al. Roux-en-Y gastric bypass in an adolescent patient with Bardet-Biedl syndrome, a monogenic obesity disorder. Obes Surg 2010;20(1):121–5.
48. Mujahid S, Huda MS, Beales P, et al. Adjustable gastric banding and sleeve gastrectomy in Bardet-Biedl syndrome. Obes Surg 2014;24(10):1746–8.
49. Cassidy SB, Driscoll DJ. Prader-Willi syndrome. Eur J Hum Genet 2009; 17(1):3–13.
50. Pedemonti B, Ceccomancini R, D'Acunti A, et al. Effectiveness of a transdisciplinary approach on hyperphagia management among patients with Prader Willi syndrome. Endocrinol Diabetes Nutr (Engl Ed). 2023;70(5):347–51.
51. Butler MG, Miller JL, Forster JL. Prader-Willi Syndrome - Clinical Genetics, Diagnosis and Treatment Approaches: An Update. Curr Pediatr Rev 2019;15(4): 207–44.
52. Heymsfield SB, Avena NM, Baier L, et al. Hyperphagia: current concepts and future directions proceedings of the 2nd international conference on hyperphagia. Obesity 2014;22(Suppl 1):S1–17.
53. Butler MG, Theodoro MF, Bittel DC, et al. Energy expenditure and physical activity in Prader-Willi syndrome: comparison with obese subjects. Am J Med Genet 2007;143A(5):449–59.
54. Bekx MT, Carrel AL, Shriver TC, et al. Decreased energy expenditure is caused by abnormal body composition in infants with Prader-Willi Syndrome. J Pediatr. Sep 2003;143(3):372–6.
55. Schoeller DA, Levitsky LL, Bandini LG, et al. Energy expenditure and body composition in Prader-Willi syndrome. Metabolism 1988;37(2):115–20.
56. Hoffman CJ, Aultman D, Pipes P. A nutrition survey of and recommendations for individuals with Prader-Willi syndrome who live in group homes. J Am Diet Assoc 1992;92(7):823–30, 833.
57. Holm VA, Pipes PL. Food and children with Prader-Willi syndrome. Am J Dis Child 1976;130(10):1063–7.
58. Lima VP, Emerich DR, Mesquita ML, et al. Nutritional intervention with hypocaloric diet for weight control in children and adolescents with Prader-Willi Syndrome. Eat Behav 2016;21:189–92.

59. Miller JL, Lynn CH, Shuster J, et al. A reduced-energy intake, well-balanced diet improves weight control in children with Prader-Willi syndrome. J Hum Nutr Diet 2013;26(1):2–9.
60. Irizarry KA, Mager DR, Triador L, et al. Hormonal and metabolic effects of carbohydrate restriction in children with Prader-Willi syndrome. Clin Endocrinol 2019;90(4):553–61.
61. Zhang C, Yin A, Li H, et al. Dietary Modulation of Gut Microbiota Contributes to Alleviation of Both Genetic and Simple Obesity in Children. EBioMedicine 2015; 2(8):968–84.
62. Akefeldt A. Water intake and risk of hyponatraemia in Prader-Willi syndrome. J Intellect Disabil Res 2009;53(6):521–8.
63. Sylvetsky AC, Figueroa J, Zimmerman T, et al. Consumption of low-calorie sweetened beverages is associated with higher total energy and sugar intake among children, NHANES 2011-2016. Pediatr Obes 2019;14(10):e12535.
64. Van Opstal AM, Hafkemeijer A, van den Berg-Huysmans AA, et al. Brain activity and connectivity changes in response to nutritive natural sugars, non-nutritive natural sugar replacements and artificial sweeteners. Nutr Neurosci 2021; 24(5):395–405.
65. Alyousif Z, Miller JL, Auger J, et al. Microbiota profile and efficacy of probiotic supplementation on laxation in adults affected by Prader-Willi Syndrome: A randomized, double-blind, crossover trial. Mol Genet Genomic Med 2020;8(12): e1535.
66. Kong XJ, Liu K, Zhuang P, et al. The Effects of Limosilactobacillus reuteri LR-99 Supplementation on Body Mass Index, Social Communication, Fine Motor Function, and Gut Microbiome Composition in Individuals with Prader-Willi Syndrome: a Randomized Double-Blinded Placebo-Controlled Trial. Probiotics Antimicrob Proteins 2021;13(6):1508–20.
67. Aycan Z, Bas VN. Prader-Willi syndrome and growth hormone deficiency. J Clin Res Pediatr Endocrinol 2014;6(2):62–7.
68. Edge R, la Fleur P, Adcock L. Human Growth Hormone Treatment for Children with Prader-Willi Syndrome: A Review of Clinical Effectiveness, Cost-Effectiveness, and Guidelines. 2018. Canadian Agency for Drugs and Technologies in Health (CADTH) Rapid response reports.
69. Luo Y, Zheng Z, Yang Y, et al. Effects of growth hormone on cognitive, motor, and behavioral development in Prader-Willi syndrome children: a meta-analysis of randomized controlled trials. Endocrine 2021;71(2):321–30.
70. Frixou M, Vlek D, Lucas-Herald AK, et al. The use of growth hormone therapy in adults with Prader-Willi syndrome: A systematic review. Clin Endocrinol 2021; 94(4):645–55.
71. Rosenberg AGW, Passone CGB, Pellikaan K, et al. Growth Hormone Treatment for Adults With Prader-Willi Syndrome: A Meta-Analysis. J Clin Endocrinol Metab 2021;106(10):3068–91.
72. Angulo M, Abuzzahab MJ, Pietropoli A, et al. Outcomes in children treated with growth hormone for Prader-Willi syndrome: data from the ANSWER Program(R) and NordiNet(R) International Outcome Study. Int J Pediatr Endocrinol 2020; 2020(1):20.
73. Irizarry KA, Miller M, Freemark M, et al. Prader Willi Syndrome: Genetics, Metabolomics, Hormonal Function, and New Approaches to Therapy. Adv Pediatr 2016;63(1):47–77.
74. Sjostrom A, Hoybye C. Twenty Years of GH Treatment in Adults with Prader-Willi Syndrome. J Clin Med 2021;10(12). https://doi.org/10.3390/jcm10122667.

75. Ng NBH, Low YW, Rajgor DD, et al. The effects of glucagon-like peptide (GLP)-1 receptor agonists on weight and glycaemic control in Prader-Willi syndrome: A systematic review. Clin Endocrinol 2022;96(2):144–54.
76. Diene G, Angulo M, Hale PM, et al. Liraglutide for Weight Management in Children and Adolescents With Prader-Willi Syndrome and Obesity. J Clin Endocrinol Metab 2022;108(1):4–12.
77. Bossart M, Wagner M, Elvert R, et al. Effects on weight loss and glycemic control with SAR441255, a potent unimolecular peptide GLP-1/GIP/GCG receptor triagonist. Cell Metab 2022;34(1):59–74.e10.
78. Goldman VE, Naguib MN, Vidmar AP. Anti-Obesity Medication Use in Children and Adolescents with Prader-Willi Syndrome: Case Review and Literature Search. J Clin Med 2021;(19):10. https://doi.org/10.3390/jcm10194540.
79. Bischof JM, Van Der Ploeg LH, Colmers WF, et al. Magel2-null mice are hyper-responsive to setmelanotide, a melanocortin 4 receptor agonist. Br J Pharmacol 2016;173(17):2614–21.
80. Young LJ, Flanagan-Cato LM. Editorial comment: oxytocin, vasopressin and social behavior. Horm Behav 2012;61(3):227–9.
81. Swaab DF, Purba JS, Hofman MA. Alterations in the hypothalamic paraventricular nucleus and its oxytocin neurons (putative satiety cells) in Prader-Willi syndrome: a study of five cases. J Clin Endocrinol Metab 1995;80(2):573–9.
82. Rice LJ, Einfeld SL, Hu N, et al. A review of clinical trials of oxytocin in Prader-Willi syndrome. Curr Opin Psychiatry 2018;31(2):123–7.
83. Einfeld SL, Smith E, McGregor IS, et al. A double-blind randomized controlled trial of oxytocin nasal spray in Prader Willi syndrome. Am J Med Genet 2014; 164A(9):2232–9.
84. Kuppens RJ, Donze SH, Hokken-Koelega AC. Promising effects of oxytocin on social and food-related behaviour in young children with Prader-Willi syndrome: a randomized, double-blind, controlled crossover trial. Clin Endocrinol 2016; 85(6):979–87.
85. Miller JL, Tamura R, Butler MG, et al. Oxytocin treatment in children with Prader-Willi syndrome: A double-blind, placebo-controlled, crossover study. Am J Med Genet 2017;173(5):1243–50.
86. Tauber M, Boulanouar K, Diene G, et al. The Use of Oxytocin to Improve Feeding and Social Skills in Infants With Prader-Willi Syndrome. Pediatrics 2017;139(2). https://doi.org/10.1542/peds.2016-2976.
87. Damen L, Grootjen LN, Juriaans AF, et al. Oxytocin in young children with Prader-Willi syndrome: Results of a randomized, double-blind, placebo-controlled, crossover trial investigating 3 months of oxytocin. Clin Endocrinol 2021;94(5):774–85.
88. Hollander E, Levine KG, Ferretti CJ, et al. Intranasal oxytocin versus placebo for hyperphagia and repetitive behaviors in children with Prader-Willi Syndrome: A randomized controlled pilot trial. J Psychiatr Res 2021;137:643–51.
89. Roof E, Deal CL, McCandless SE, et al. Intranasal Carbetocin Reduces Hyperphagia, Anxiousness and Distress in Prader-Willi Syndrome: CARE-PWS Phase 3 Trial. J Clin Endocrinol Metab 2023. https://doi.org/10.1210/clinem/dgad015.
90. Kuppens RJ, Diene G, Bakker NE, et al. Elevated ratio of acylated to unacylated ghrelin in children and young adults with Prader-Willi syndrome. Endocrine 2015;50(3):633–42.
91. Allas S, Caixas A, Poitou C, et al. AZP-531, an unacylated ghrelin analog, improves food-related behavior in patients with Prader-Willi syndrome: A randomized placebo-controlled trial. PLoS One 2018;13(1):e0190849.

92. Mahmoud R, Kimonis V, Butler MG. Clinical Trials in Prader-Willi Syndrome: A Review. Int J Mol Sci 2023;24(3). https://doi.org/10.3390/ijms24032150.
93. Miller JL, Lacroix A, Bird LM, et al. The Efficacy, Safety, and Pharmacology of a Ghrelin O-Acyltransferase Inhibitor for the Treatment of Prader-Willi Syndrome. J Clin Endocrinol Metab 2022. https://doi.org/10.1210/clinem/dgac105.
94. Kimonis V, Surampalli A, Wencel M, et al. A randomized pilot efficacy and safety trial of diazoxide choline controlled-release in patients with Prader-Willi syndrome. PLoS One 2019;14(9):e0221615.
95. Miller JL, Gevers E, Bridges N, et al. Diazoxide Choline Extended-Release Tablet in People With Prader-Willi Syndrome: A Double-Blind, Placebo-Controlled Trial. J Clin Endocrinol Metab 2023;108(7):1676–85.
96. White HM, Acton AJ, Considine RV. The angiogenic inhibitor TNP-470 decreases caloric intake and weight gain in high-fat fed mice. Obesity 2012;20(10):2003–9.
97. Rupnick MA, Panigrahy D, Zhang CY, et al. Adipose tissue mass can be regulated through the vasculature. Proc Natl Acad Sci U S A 2002;99(16):10730–5.
98. Brakenhielm E, Cao R, Gao B, et al. Angiogenesis inhibitor, TNP-470, prevents diet-induced and genetic obesity in mice. Circ Res 2004;94(12):1579–88.
99. McCandless SE, Yanovski JA, Miller J, et al. Effects of MetAP2 inhibition on hyperphagia and body weight in Prader-Willi syndrome: A randomized, double-blind, placebo-controlled trial. Diabetes Obes Metab 2017;19(12):1751–61.
100. Saniona Receives U.S. FDA Orphan Drug Designation for Tesomet in Prader-Willi Syndrome. Press Release on March 3, 2021. Available at: https://www.globenewswire.com/news-release/2021/03/03/2186073/0/en/Saniona-Receives-U-S-FDA-Orphan-Drug-Designation-for-Tesomet-in-Prader-Willi-Syndrome.html Accessed September 22, 2023.
101. Huynh K, Klose M, Krogsgaard K, et al. Randomized controlled trial of Tesomet for weight loss in hypothalamic obesity. Eur J Endocrinol 2022;186(6):687–700.
102. Nolan BJ, Proietto J, Sumithran P. Intensive management of obesity in people with Prader-Willi syndrome. Endocrine 2022;77(1):57–62.
103. Knani I, Earley BJ, Udi S, et al. Targeting the endocannabinoid/CB1 receptor system for treating obesity in Prader-Willi syndrome. Mol Metab 2016;5(12):1187–99.
104. Motaghedi R, Lipman EG, Hogg JE, et al. Psychiatric adverse effects of rimonobant in adults with Prader Willi syndrome. Eur J Med Genet 2011;54(1):14–8.
105. Wolfe G, Salehi V, Browne A, et al. Metabolic and bariatric surgery for obesity in Prader Willi syndrome: systematic review and meta-analysis. Surg Obes Relat Dis 2023. https://doi.org/10.1016/j.soard.2023.01.017.
106. Queen NJ, Zou X, Anderson JM, et al. Hypothalamic AAV-BDNF gene therapy improves metabolic function and behavior in the Magel2-null mouse model of Prader-Willi syndrome. Mol Ther Methods Clin Dev 2022;27:131–48.
107. Kaur Y, de Souza RJ, Gibson WT, et al. A systematic review of genetic syndromes with obesity. Obes Rev 2017;18(6):603–34.

Management of Medication-Induced Weight Gain

Sarah R. Barenbaum, MD[a,*], Rekha B. Kumar, MD, MS[b], Louis J. Aronne, MD[a]

KEYWORDS

- Medication-induced weight gain • Iatrogenic obesity • Medication-induced obesity
- Obesity • Treatment of iatrogenic obesity
- Treatment of medication-induced weight gain

KEY POINTS

- Medication-induced weight gain is common and may be preventable.
- Prescribe medications that are weight neutral or that lead to weight loss, when possible.
- When prescribing medications that cause weight gain, use the lowest effective dose for the shortest amount of time in order to mitigate weight gain.

INTRODUCTION

A plethora of commonly prescribed medications can lead to weight gain or can make it difficult for patients to lose weight.[1] It is imperative for health-care providers to know which medications fall into these categories because medication-induced obesity is potentially avoidable with the use of weight-neutral or weight-losing medications.[2] Additionally, drug-induced weight gain can lead to nonadherence with the prescribed medication and may lead to worsening of obesity-related comorbidities. When prescribing a new medication or considering a change, the provider should take the patients' weight status and risk factors for metabolic disease into consideration versus the benefits of the new pharmacotherapy. Common classes of medications that lead to weight gain include antidiabetes, psychotropic medications (including antidepressants, antianxiety, antipsychotics, and mood stabilizers), anticonvulsants, antihypertensives, antihistamines, contraceptives, steroids, and hormones. This review will focus on the common classes of medications that can lead to weight gain and alternative medications to consider (summarized in **Table 1**) and treatment strategies for medication-induced weight gain.

[a] Division of Endocrinology, Diabetes & Metabolism, NewYork-Presbyterian Hospital/ Weill Cornell Medical College, Comprehensive Weight Control Center, 1305 York Avenue, 4th Floor, New York, NY 10021, USA; [b] Iris Cantor Women's Health Center, Endocrinology & Internal Medicine, 425 East 61st Street, Fl 11, New York, NY 10065, USA
* Corresponding author.
E-mail address: srb9023@med.cornell.edu

Gastroenterol Clin N Am 52 (2023) 751–760
https://doi.org/10.1016/j.gtc.2023.08.006

Table 1
Medications that cause weight gain and alternatives to consider

Weight Gain	Weight Neutral	Weight Loss
Antidiabetic medications Insulin Sulfonylureas Thiazolidinediones	DPP-4 inhibitors Alpha-glucosidase inhibitors	Metformin Tirzepatide GLP-1 agonists SGLT2 inhibitors Pramlintide
Antidepressants SSRIs (except fluoxetine, sertraline), MAOIs, TCAs, and mirtazapine	Fluoxetine, sertraline, and SNRIs	Bupropion
Antipsychotics Typical and atypical antipsychotics particularly risperidone, quetiapine, clozapine, and olanzapine	Lurasidone and ziprasidone	
Mood stabilizers Lithium		Topiramate and zonisamide
Antiepileptics Gabapentin, pregabalin, carbamazepine, and valproic acid	Lamotrigine, levetiracetam, and phenytoin	Topiramate and zonisamide
Antihypertensives β-blockers (atenolol, metoprolol, nadolol, and propranolol) α-blockers	β-blockers (carvedilol and nebivolol) ACE inhibitors ARB inhibitors CCBs Thiazides	
Antihistamines Sedating and nonsedating antihistamines	Loratadine	
Steroids Glucocorticoids Corticosteroids	DMARDs	
Contraceptives Progesterone implants and hormonal IUD		Copper IUD and barrier methods

Abbreviations: ACE, angiotensin-converting enzyme; ARB, angiotensin receptor blockers; CCBs, calcium channel blockers; DMARDs, disease-modifying antirheumatic drugs; DPP-4, dipeptidyl peptidase IV; GLP-1, Glucagon-like peptide-1; MAOIs, monoamine oxidase inhibitors; SGLT2, Sodium-glucose cotransporter; SNRIs, serotonin and norepinephrine reuptake inhibitors; SSRIs, selective serotonin reuptake inhibitors; TCAs, tricyclic antidepressants.

ANTIDIABETES MEDICATIONS

Several medications used to treat diabetes are associated with weight gain, particularly insulin, sulfonylureas, and other insulin secretagogues.[3] These medications are associated with as much weight gain as 10 kg in 3 to 6 months after initiating treatment.[4]

Metformin is a first-line treatment of type 2 diabetes and is one of the most commonly prescribed antidiabetes medications due to its efficacy, durability and safety profile, low risk of hypoglycemia, and ability to promote modest weight loss.[5] Metformin can lead to weight loss through a variety of mechanisms, including increasing insulin sensitivity, decreasing intestinal absorption of glucose, and decreasing hepatic gluconeogenesis. It may also enhance energy metabolism by promoting a catabolic state via increasing phosphorylation of adenosine monophosphate (AMP)-activated protein kinase. This activation leads to a shift away from lipid accretion and storage, resulting in weight loss.[6] In addition, in rat models, metformin has been shown to increase leptin sensitivity and to decrease leptin resistance, and in rodent models, it has been shown to increase circulating levels of GDF15, which suppresses appetite and increases energy expenditure.[7–9]

Participants in the Diabetes Prevention Program with overweight and obesity were randomized to lifestyle modifications with metformin 850 mg twice daily versus standard lifestyle with placebo. At 1-year and 2-years, the total body weight was significantly reduced in the metformin group (2.7% vs 0.43%, and 2.1% vs 0.02%, respectively), and long-term follow-up data illustrated that the metformin group-maintained weight loss of 6.2% between years 6 and 15 versus 2.8% weight loss in the placebo group.[10,11]

Glucagon-like peptide-1 (GLP-1) agonists, another class of medications used to treat diabetes, promote weight loss. Human GLP-1 is an incretin hormone that is secreted in the gut in response to nutrients. There are GLP-1 receptors throughout the body, and binding to them helps to improve glycemic control and to promote weight loss through a variety of mechanisms. When GLP-1 binds to GLP-1 receptors in the gut it leads to a reduction in gastric emptying and a subsequent reduction in food intake. GLP-1 also binds to receptors in the brain which helps to regulate appetite. GLP-1 additionally leads to a peripheral stimulation of insulin and reduction in glucagon. In the trials for the treatment of diabetes, patients on semaglutide 0.5 mg and 1.0 mg lost 3.5 kg to 4.6 kg and 4.5 kg to 6.5 kg, respectively, versus baseline.[12] In a phase 3b trial comparing semaglutide 1.0 mg to semaglutide 2.0 mg, at week 40, mean changes in bodyweight were −6.0 kg versus −6.9 kg, respectively.[13] Two GLP-1 agonists, liraglutide 3.0 mg and semaglutide 2.4 mg, are approved by the Food and Drug Administration (FDA) for the treatment of overweight and obesity. In the clinical trials at 56 weeks, participants on liraglutide 3.0 mg daily lost 8.0% of their total body weight versus 2.6% in the placebo group.[14] At 68 weeks on semaglutide 2.4 mg weekly, participants lost 14.9% of their total body weight versus 2.4% on placebo.[15]

Tirzepatide, the first GLP-1 and glucose-dependent insulinotropic polypeptide (GIP) dual agonist, was approved by the FDA in 2022 for the treatment of diabetes, also promotes significant weight loss. Along with GLP-1, GIP enhances postprandial insulin secretion in a glucose-dependent manner. It also stimulates glucagon during hypoglycemia and positively influences lipid homeostasis.[16] It is hypothesized that GIP may lead to weight loss by acting centrally to potentiate the GLP-1-induced reduction in food intake, and animal models have shown that GIP may act centrally on satiety centers. Finally, the dual agonism may lead to greater improvement in both weight and glucose control than a GLP-1 alone.[16,17] In the phase III trials for the treatment of diabetes, there was a dose-dependent reduction in weight and subjects lost 7 to 9.5 kg on tirzepatide. In the ongoing phase III clinical weight-loss trials, average weight loss at 72 weeks was 20.9% on the maximum dose of tirzepatide versus 3.1% on placebo.[18]

Sodium-glucose cotransporter 2 (SGLT2 inhibitors) are expressed in the proximal tubule of the kidney and mediate the reabsorption of glucose. SGLT2 inhibitors therefore promote the renal excretion of glucose, which leads to improved glycemic control. Through this mechanism SGLT2 inhibitors also contribute to modest weight loss and can lower blood pressure. In most studies, SGLT-2 inhibitors have led to modest weight loss (around 1–3 kg).[19]

Pramlintide is an amylin analog used to treat insulin dependent type 1 and type 2 diabetes. Amylin is an amino acid peptide that is stored in the pancreatic beta cells and cosecreted with insulin. Amylin slows gastric emptying, reduces food intake, slows the increase of postprandial glucagon, and may increase satiety.[20,21] Pramlintide overall leads to better glucose regulation and reduction in exogenous insulin and is associated with weight loss.

Dipeptidyl peptidase IV (DPP-4) inhibitors seem to be weight neutral or may lead to minimal weight change. Alpha-glucosidase inhibitors (such as miglitol or acarbose) may also be weight neutral or lead to a minimal change in weight.[22,23]

The 2016 Endocrine Society Clinical Practice Guidelines on the pharmacologic management of obesity recommend using weight-losing and weight-neutral medications as the first-line and second-line agents in the management of type 2 diabetes in patients with overweight and obesity. In addition, they recommend treating individuals who have both obesity and type 2 diabetes who require insulin with at least one of either metformin, a GLP-1 agonist or pramlintide to reduce the weight gain associated with insulin. They also recommend initiating treatment with basal insulin instead of insulin alone.[4]

The 2022 American Association of Clinical Endocrinologists Clinical Practice Guidelines on diabetes recommend that the initiation of antidiabetes medications should be prescribed based on evidence that the pharmacotherapy improves glycemic control, avoids hypoglycemia and weight gain, and reduces cardio-renal risk. The guidelines recommend that the therapy should be individualized based on the level of glycemia, risk factors, and comorbidities. The new algorithm suggests that although metformin is often preferred as initial monotherapy, other agents may be more appropriate as initial therapy or in addition to metformin if a patient has additional comorbidities, such as obesity, cardiovascular disease, nonalcoholic fatty liver disease, and chronic kidney disease, independent of the glucose-lowering affects. When insulin is required, these guidelines also recommend starting with long-acting insulin, and addition of a GLP-1 before adding meal-time insulin.[24]

Therefore, although several medications used to treat diabetes lead to weight gain, there are many options that are weight neutral or that lead to weight loss. As with all medications, it is not always possible to start with a medication that falls into these categories, for example, if a patient requires insulin. However, when patients with overweight or obesity do require insulin, consider adding another first-line or second-line medication that will help reduce insulin requirements to mitigate weight gain and/or lead to weight loss.

PSYCHOTROPIC MEDICATIONS

Prescriptions for psychotropic medications, particularly antidepressants, have increased significantly during the past few decades.[25] Many commonly prescribed psychotropic medications lead to weight gain. These include antidepressants, antipsychotics, and mood stabilizers.[2] Psychotropic medications vary widely in regard to weight-gaining potential, and it can depend on length of therapy.[26] In addition, the influence of the pharmacotherapy itself can be hard to quantify because weight gain in patients with psychiatric conditions can be multifactorial and depression itself is characterized by changes in energy, appetite, and physical activity.[27] Finally individual response may vary; although one medication will cause weight gain in one individual, it may lead to weight loss in another. Weight gain with a medication is particularly concerning in that, aside from obvious health risks associated with overweight and obesity, it may lead to patient noncompliance with psychotropic medications that can have serious mental health consequences.

Antidepressants

Antidepressants can lead to variable but significant weight gain. Among the antidepressants, monoamine oxidase inhibitors (MAOIs), selective serotonin reuptake inhibitors (SSRIs), tricyclic antidepressants (TCAs), and mirtazapine have been shown to have the greatest risk of weight gain. Although several mechanisms are likely present, antidepressants may induce weight gain by acting centrally as an orexigenic agent, increasing appetite and food intake.[28]

One meta-analysis,[27] which looked at 116 studies found that amitriptyline was the most potent weight-gaining agent of the TCAs and was significantly associated with weight gain both in the acute treatment (4–12 weeks) and maintenance periods (>4 months). Mirtazapine and nortriptyline were also significantly associated with weight gain during the acute and long-term treatment period. Of the SSRIs, paroxetine was found to lead to the greatest long-term increases in body weight. Some SSRIs, such as fluoxetine and sertraline, were associated with weight loss in the acute treatment phase and then weight neutrality after. Finally bupropion was the only antidepressant noted to lead to weight loss, which was sustained over time.

Bupropion, a dopamine and norepinephrine reuptake inhibitor, is the only antidepressant consistently associated with weight loss.[29] It has been shown to decrease body weight by reducing food cravings and suppressing appetite.[30] Bupropion was initially FDA-approved for the treatment of depression and then as a smoking cessation aide. It was later approved by the FDA as a combination medication of bupropion sustained release and naltrexone for the treatment of chronic weight management. Bupropion therefore may be a suitable antidepressant option for those struggling with weight, or for those in whom weight gain is a concern, although it is not appropriate for all patients with depression because it is activating and therefore can exacerbate anxiety or may be inappropriate for a patient with bipolar disorder.

Ultimately the choice of which antidepressant to use must be based on what is best for the patient because there are different classes of antidepressants used for different types of depression. The few antidepressants which are weight neutral or weight losing are not appropriate for all patients with depression. When an antidepressant is indicated, a shared decision-making process should be considered with the patient, and patients should be counseled on the potential for weight gain with certain agents. If there is significant weight gain early in treatment, physicians should consider whether alternative agents may be appropriate. When possible, physicians should reevaluate the success of the medication and the continued need for it on regular intervals.

Antipsychotics

Antipsychotics are a class of psychotropic medications that are associated with significant weight gain, along with glucose dysregulation and dyslipidemia.[31,32] The mechanism is thought to be due to an interaction with serotonergic, dopaminergic, adrenergic, and histaminergic systems, which has a central influence on energy homeostasis, appetite, and satiety.[33] Risperidone, quetiapine, clozapine, and olanzapine are associated with weight gain across multiple studies.[32,34] A meta-analysis which compared 15 antipsychotic medications and looked at 212 trials found that ziprasidone and lurasidone did not produce more weight gain than placebo.[35]

A meta-analysis, which looked at the use of augmentation of antipsychotics in patients with schizophrenia with other medications such as topiramate, an antiepileptic used off-label as a mood stabilizer, found that augmentation may lead to an improvement in psychiatric function and weight loss.[36] Although this strategy will not work with all patients, a lower dose of antipsychotic medication may be achieved when augmented with another agent. Another strategy that may be tried is treatment with metformin. Metformin may help to reduce the effects of weight gain that are associated with antipsychotic use.[5]

ANTICONVULSANTS

Anticonvulsants often cause weight gain. In particular, gabapentin, pregabalin, carbamazepine, and valproic acid are associated with weight gain.[37] Valproic acid may lead to weight gain by causing leptin resistance, although other proposed mechanisms are multifactorial and include hypothalamic dysfunction, an effect on adipokines, insulin resistance, genetic susceptibility, and hyperinsulinemia.[38,39] Meanwhile, lamotrigine, phenytoin, and levetiracetam are considered weight neutral.[38] Topiramate and zonisamide are consistently associated with weight loss.[38] Aside from being FDA-approved as an anticonvulsant, topiramate is also FDA-approved for migraines and for chronic weight management in a combination pill with phentermine. Topiramate is used off label as a mood stabilizer, therefore, if appropriate it may be considered as alternatives to medications such as lithium or antipsychotics, which may cause weight gain.

ANTIHYPERTENSIVES

Beta-blockers (β-blockers) are a commonly used antihypertensive medication and have additional benefits of reducing overall cardiovascular morbidity and mortality.[40] Unfortunately, many β-blockers are associated with the development of dyslipidemia and insulin resistance and may decrease metabolic rate by as much as 12%, leading to weight gain.[41,42] The amount of weight gain due to β-blockers is variable and individualized but can be significant.

Interestingly, not all β-blockers are associated with weight gain. Selective β-blockers that have a vasodilating component, such as carvedilol and nebivolol, seem to have less of an influence on lipids, insulin, metabolic rate, and weight gain.[43] The pathophysiologic reason for this is not entirely clear.

When treating patients for hypertension, if a patient would benefit from β-blockers, particularly patients with coronary artery disease, heart failure, or an arrhythmia, using carvedilol or nebivolol is preferable from a weight standpoint if they are tolerated and not contraindicated for another reason. Alternatively, there are many other classes of antihypertensives that are not associated with weight gain including angiotensin-converting enzyme (ACE) inhibitors, angiotensin receptor blockers (ARB) inhibitors, and calcium channel blockers (CCBs).[43] These medications are preferable from a weight-standpoint.

ANTIHISTAMINES

Antihistamines are frequently prescribed but also available over the counter and may cause considerable weight gain. In animal studies, histamine itself reduced food intake, whereas antihistamines increased food intake. In humans, antihistamines may lead to weight gain by stimulating appetite.[44] The amount of weight gain may be proportional to the potency of the antihistamine; therefore, it is suggested that patients use antihistamines that are less centrally acting and milder when possible.[4] Patients may forget to mention the antihistamine they are taking over the counter (for allergies, as part of sleep-aids, and so forth), which is why a thorough medication reconciliation is important at every patient encounter. If patients are purchasing them over the counter (as opposed to prescribed by a provider), encourage the patient to use the medication as less as necessary because they can cause weight gain.

CONTRACEPTIVES, HORMONES, STEROIDS

Historically, oral contraceptive pills contained high doses of both progestin and estrogen. High doses of estrogen can lead to weight gain via fluid retention and increased appetite. Newer oral contraceptive pills, however, contain lower doses of hormones and are less likely to lead to weight gain, although they still can. Progesterone implants, including progesterone intrauterine devices (IUDs) can lead to weight gain. One systematic review of 24 studies of depot medroxyprogesterone acetate (DMPA) found that the most frequently reported side effect was weight gain and reported an association between DMPA use and weight gain, including increased body fat mass.[45] If appropriate, barrier methods or a copper IUDs are forms of nonhormonal birth control that will not lead to weight gain.

Steroids can also cause significant weight gain. One survey study of 2446 participants on glucocorticoids found that weight gain was the most common self-reported adverse event (70% of individuals).[46] For patients with inflammatory conditions that require treatment, disease-modifying antirheumatic drugs (DMARDs) are preferable when possible.

DISCUSSION

Many physicians are unaware of the extreme consequences that medication-induced weight gain can have—namely development or exacerbation of obesity and the many obesity-related comorbidities. The best way to treat medication-induced weight gain is to prevent it from occurring. This requires awareness of which medications are more likely to lead to weight gain, which medications are weight neutral, and which medications can lead to weight loss. Providers should complete a thorough medication reconciliation when meeting with patients, specifically inquiring about over-the-counter medications because patients may forget to report them, and they can include medications such as a daily antihistamine (or sleep aid, which may include an antihistamine).

It not always possible or appropriate to avoid medications that cause weight gain especially if that medication is best practice for the patient's condition. When medications that cause weight gain are necessary, use a shared decision-making model with patients and fully inform them of the potential for weight gain. If possible, use the lowest dose of a medication for the shortest period of time because this can mitigate weight gain. If appropriate, try to lower the dose of medication by augmenting with a second medication that is weight neutral or weight losing.

When treating medication-induced weight gain, do not discontinue or change an offending medication without first discussing whether it is appropriate with the prescribing provider. If long-term use of a weight-promoting medication is required, or if a patient rapidly gains weight when initiating a necessary treatment, monitor closely for weight gain and consider referring to an obesity medicine specialist for treatment.

DISCLOSURE

S.R. Barenbaum reports no disclosures. R.B. Kumar is the Chief Medical Officer of Found, a digital weight care platform (executive position and equity ownership). She also reports receiving consulting fees from Eli Lilly, Novo Nordisk, and Gelesis. She is a shareholder in Vivus and Myos Corp. Dr L.J. Aronne reports receiving consulting fees from/and serving on advisory boards for Allurion, Altimmune, Atria, Gelesis, Jamieson Wellness, Janssen Pharmaceuticals, Jazz Pharmaceuticals, Novo Nordisk, Pfizer, Optum, Eli Lilly, Senda Biosciences, and Versanis; receiving research funding from Allurion, AstraZeneca, United Kingdom, Gelesis, Janssen Pharmaceuticals, United States Novo Nordisk, Denmark and Eli Lilly & Co, United States; having equity interests in Allurion, ERX Pharmaceuticals, Gelesis, Intellihealth, Jamieson Wellness and Myos Corp; and serving on a board of directors for ERX Pharmaceuticals, Intellihealth, and Jamieson Wellness.

REFERENCES

1. Apovian C, Aronne L, Barenbaum S. Clinical management of obesity. 2nd edition. West Islip, NY: Professional Communications, Inc.; 2022.
2. Domecq JP, Prutsky G, Leppin A, et al. Clinical review: Drugs commonly associated with weight change: a systematic review and meta-analysis. J Clin Endocrinol Metab 2015;100(2):363–70.
3. Phung OJ, Scholle JM, Talwar M, et al. Effect of noninsulin antidiabetic drugs added to metformin therapy on glycemic control, weight gain, and hypoglycemia in type 2 diabetes. JAMA 2010;303:1410–8.
4. Apovian CM, Aronne LJ, Bessesen DH, et al. Pharmacological management of obesity: an endocrine Society clinical practice guideline. J Clin Endocrinol Metab 2015;100(2):342–62.
5. Igel LI, Sinha A, Saunders KH, et al. Metformin: an Old Therapy that Deserves a New Indication for the Treatment of Obesity. Curr Atheroscler Rep 2016;18(4):16.
6. Hawley SA, Gadalla AE, Olsen GS, et al. The antidiabetic drug metformin activates the AMP-activated protein kinase cascade via an adenine nucleotide-independent mechanism. Diabetes 2002;51(8):2420–5.
7. Hostalek U, Gwilt M, Hildemann S. Therapeutic Use of Metformin in Prediabetes and Diabetes Prevention. Drugs 2015;75(10):1071–94.
8. Coll AP, Chen M, Taskar P, et al. GDF15 mediates the effects of metformin on body weight and energy balance. Nature 2020;578(2295):444–8.
9. Kim YW, Kim JY, Park YH, et al. Metformin restores leptin sensitivity in high-fat-fed obese rats with leptin resistance. Diabetes 2006;55(3):716–24.
10. Diabetes Prevention Program Research Group. 10-year follow-up of diabetes incidence and weight loss in the Diabetes Prevention Program Outcomes Study. Lancet 2009;374(9702):1677–86.
11. Apolzan JW, Venditti EM, Edelstein SL, et al. Long-Term Weight Loss With Metformin or Lifestyle Intervention in the Diabetes Prevention Program Outcomes Study. Ann Intern Med 2019;170(10):682–90.
12. Goldenberg R, Steen O. Semaglutide: Review and Place in Therapy for Adults With Type 2 Diabetes. Can J Diabetes 2019;43(2):136–45.
13. Frias J, Auerbach P, Bajaj H, et al. Efficacy and safety of once-weekly semaglutide 2.0 mg versus 1.0 mg in patients with type 2 diabetes (SUSTAIN FORTE): a double-blind, randomized, phase 3B trial. Lancet Diabetes Endocrinol 2021;9: 563–74.

14. Pi-Sunyer X, Astrup A, Fujioka K, et al. A Randomized, Controlled Trial of 3.0 mg of Liraglutide in Weight Management. N Engl J Med 2015;373(1):11–22.
15. Wilding J, Batterham R, Calanna S, et al. Once-weekly Semaglutide in Adults with Overweight or Obesity. N Engl J Med 2021;384(11):989–1002.
16. Rosenstock J, Wysham C, Frias J, et al. Efficacy and safety of a novel dual GIP and GLP-1 receptor agonist tirzepatide in patients with type 2 diabetes (SURPASS-1): a double-blind, randomised, phase 3 trial. Lancet 2021;398(10295): 143–55.
17. Frias J, Davies M, Rosenstock J, et al. Tirzepatide versus Semaglutide Once Weekly in Patients with Type 2 Diabetes. N Engl J Med 2021;385(6):503–15.
18. Jastreboff A, Aronne L, Ahmad N, et al. Tirzepatide Once Weekly for the Treatment of Obesity. N Engl J Med 2022;387(3):205–16.
19. Lee PC, Ganguly S, Goh SY. Weight loss associated with sodium-glucose cotransporter-2 inhibition: a review of evidence and underlying mechanisms. Obes Rev 2018;19(12):1630–41.
20. Ratner R, Want L, Fineman M. Adjunctive Therapy with the Amylin Analogue Pramlintide Leads to a Combined Improvement in Glycemic and Weight Control in Insulin-Treated Subjects with Type 2 Diabetes. Diabetes Technol Therapeut 2002;4(1):51–61.
21. Riddle M, Frias J, Zhang B, et al. Pramlintide improved glycemic control and reduced weight in patients with type 2 diabetes using basal insulin. Diabetes Care 2007;30(11):2794–9.
22. Lee A, Patrick P, Wishart J, et al. The effects of miglitol on glucagon-like peptide-1 secretion and appetite sensations in obese type 2 diabetics. Diabetes Obes Metab 2002;4(5):329–35.
23. van de Laar FA, Lucassen PL, Akkermans RP, et al. Alpha-glucosidase inhibitors for patients with type 2 diabetes: results from a Cochrane systematic review and meta-analysis. Diabetes Care 2005;28(1):154–63.
24. Blonde L, Umpierrez GE, Reddy SS, et al. American Association of Clinical Endocrinology Clinical Practice Guideline: Developing a Diabetes Mellitus Comprehensive Care Plan-2022 Update. Endocr Pract 2022;28(10):923–1049.
25. Serretti A, Porcelli S. Antidepressant induced weight gain. BMJ 2018;361:1–2.
26. Saunders KH, Igel LI, Shukla AP, et al. Drug-induced weight gain: Rethinking our choices. J Fam Pract 2016;65(11):780–2, 784-786,788.
27. Serretti A, Mandelli L. Antidepressants and Body Weight: A Comprehensive Review and Meta-Analysis. J Clin Psychiatry 2010;71(10):1259–72.
28. Meister B. Neurotransmitters in key neurons of the hypothalamus that regulate feeding behavior and body weight. Physiol Behav 2007;92(1–2):263–71.
29. Gadde KM, Xiong GL. Bupropion for weight reduction. Expert Rev Neurother 2007;7:17–24.
30. Gadde KM, Parker CB, Maner LG, et al. Bupropion for weight loss: An investigation of efficacy and tolerability in overweight and obese women. Obes Res 2001; 9:544–51.
31. Lieberman JA, Stroup TS, McEvoy JP, et al. Effectiveness of antipsychotic drugs in patients with chronic schizophrenia. N Engl J Med 2005;353:1209–23.
32. Hasnain M, Vieweg WVR, Fredrickson SK. Metformin for atypical antipsychotic-induced weight gain and glucose metabolism dysreg- ulation: review of the literature and clinical suggestions—ProQuest. CNS Drugs 2010;24(3):193–206.
33. Singh A, Ricardo-Silgado M, Bielinski S, et al. Pharmacogenomics of Medication-Induced Weight Gain and Antiobesity Medications. Obesity 2021;29:265–73.

34. Fiedorowicz JG, Miller DD, Bishop JR, et al. Systematic review and meta-analysis of pharmacological interventions for weight gain from antipsychotics and mood stabilizers. Curr Psychiatry Rev 2012;8(1):25–36.
35. Leucht S, Cipriani A, Spineli L, et al. Comparative efficacy and tolerability of 15 antipsychotic drugs in schizophrenia: a multiple-treatments meta-analysis. Lancet 2013;382(9896):951–62.
36. Correll C, Maayan L, Kane J, et al. Efficacy for Psychopathology and Body Weight and Safety of Topiramate-Antipsychotic Cotreatment in Patients With Schizophrenia Spectrum Disorders: Results From a Meta-Analysis of Randomized Controlled Trials. J Clin Psychiatry 2016;77(6):e746.
37. Gaspari CN, Guerreiro CA. Modification in body weight associated with antiepileptic drugs. Arq Neuropsiquiatr 2010;68:277–81.
38. Kilic H, Demirel A, Uysal S. The effects of valproate on serum leptin, insulin, and lipid levels in epileptic children. Pediatric International 2021;63:1351–6.
39. Verrotti A, D'Egidio C, Mohn A, et al. Weight gain following treatment with valproic acid: pathogenetic mechanisms and clinical implications. Obes Rev 2011;12: e32–43.
40. Sharma AM, Pischon T, Hardt S, et al. Hypothesis: Beta-adrenergic receptor blockers and weight gain: A systematic analysis. Hypertension 2001;37(2):250–4.
41. Pischon T, Sharma AM. Use of beta-blockers in obesity hypertension: potential role of weight gain. Obes Rev 2001;2(4):275–80.
42. Messerli FH, Bell DS, Fonseca V, et al. Body weight changes with beta-blocker use: results from GEMINI. Am J Med 2007;120(7):610–5.
43. Wing LM, Reid CM, Ryan P, et al. Second Australian National Blood Pressure Study Group. A Comparison of outcomes with angiotensin- converting enzyme inhibitors and diuretics for hypertension in the elderly. N Engl J Med 2003; 348(7):583–92.
44. Ratliff JC, Barber JA, Palmese LB, et al. Association of prescription H1 antihistamine use with obesity: results from the National Health and Nutrition Examination Survey. Obesity 2010;18(12):2398–400.
45. Dianat S, Fox E, Ahrens KA, et al. Side Effects and Health Benefits of Depot Medroxyprogesterone Acetate: A Systematic Review. Obstet Gynecol 2019;133:332.
46. Curtis J, Westfall A, Allison J, et al. Population-Based Assessment of Adverse Events Associated With Long-Term Glucocorticoid Use. Arthritis Rheum 2006; 55(3):420–6.

Language Frames and Shapes the Response to Obesity

Theodore K. Kyle, RPh, MBA[a,*], Scott Kahan, MD, MPH[b], Joe Nadglowski, BS[c]

KEYWORDS

- Obesity • Health stigma • Implicit bias • Health communication
- Stigmatizing language • Public perceptions • Barriers to health

KEY POINTS

- Implicit bias about obesity and people who live with it can be an impediment to individual and public health.
- Language serves an important role in shaping the public understanding of obesity.
- Language that promotes misinformation, stigma, and ineffective approaches to obesity can thus contribute to health risks.
- Shaping a more effective response to obesity can start with the careful use of language that frames obesity in ways that are person centered, scientifically accurate, easily understood, and limits risk of bias.

INTRODUCTION

Ten years have passed since the American Medical Association resolved that obesity is a complex chronic disease.[1] Since then, much has changed in the response to medical and public health challenges that obesity presents. Research from Project Implicit suggests that explicit weight bias has become less prevalent but implicit weight bias increased through 2010 and then remained persistently high.[2] Notably, weight bias stands out in this research from other forms of implicit bias that declined between 2007 and 2020.

Implicit bias is an impediment to the health of people living with obesity because it contributes to poorer quality of medical care. Additionally, people with obesity often avoid health-care settings due to experiences of humiliation, stress, and feeling dismissed

[a] ConscienHealth, 2270 Country Club Drive, Pittsburgh, PA 15241, USA; [b] George Washington University School of Medicine, National Center for Weight and Wellness, 1020 19th Street, Northwest, Washington, DC 20036, USA; [c] Obesity Action Coalition, 4511 N Himes Avenue, Tampa, FL 33614, USA
* Corresponding author.
E-mail address: ted.kyle@conscienhealth.org

https://doi.org/10.1016/j.gtc.2023.09.002

when seeking medical care. Too often, their experiences are more demeaning than helpful with their goals for seeking health.

Language serves as an important signal of the bias and stigma connected to the diagnosis of obesity. We use words to define what obesity is and what it is not. Historically, the language used to describe weight gain and obesity implied that these are simple behavioral problems resulting from poor lifestyle choices, to be remedied with better choices and better behavior. Even as the scientific understanding of the biological basis for obesity has improved, remnants of language implying obesity is simply an issue of personal responsibility, not a biological problem, remain—even in scientific literature.

Because of the importance of language for shaping the public and medical understanding of obesity, attention to the subtleties of language used to describe obesity, including its causes, treatment, and prevention, is important for developing more effective responses to this disease and reducing the burden it causes for individual and public health.

A STIGMATIZED DIAGNOSIS

People living with obesity report experiencing bias and stigma linked to their condition across numerous settings, including family and personal relationships, education, employment, and health care.[3] The social stigma of obesity interferes with quality of life, educational attainment, economic security, and access to effective health care.

Research on the explicit dehumanization of persons with obesity is helpful for understanding the overwhelming nature of stigma attached to a diagnosis of obesity. In 4 distinct studies, Kersbergen and Robinson found evidence for blatant dehumanization of individuals living with obesity:

"Across multiple studies, people with obesity were rated as less evolved and less human than people without obesity. This blatant dehumanization of those with obesity was evident among participants from the United States, the United Kingdom, and India and was associated with greater support for policies that discriminate against people with obesity."[4]

Although explicit weight bias has become less prevalent, evidence suggests that implicit bias has increased. In an analysis of data from Project Implicit, Charlesworth and Banaji found declining trends in explicit bias for sexual identity, race, skin tone, age, disability, and weight between 2007 and 2020. They also found that implicit bias for sexuality, race, and skin tone also declined. Implicit bias for age and disability did not change significantly. However, for weight alone, implicit bias increased and then remained high[2] (**Fig. 1**).

Much of the stigma associated with a diagnosis of obesity stems from a fundamental misunderstanding of this complex, chronic disease. Obesity has a largely genetic and physiologic basis. Behaviors associated with obesity can be the result of physiologic hunger and because of this a primary cause of obesity may be physiologic hunger, rather than behaviors that hunger prompts. However, the public and many health professionals persist in framing obesity as simply the result of unhealthy behaviors and poor personal choices.

Thus, the language we use to frame discourse about obesity can either perpetuate those misperceptions or alternately help to shape more accurate perceptions. Language is also an important tool for expressing implicit bias in social interactions and in clinical care.[5] Over time, the words we use not only reflect the attitudes we have but may also shape implicit beliefs.[6] Stigmatizing language such as "morbidly obese"[7] or "recidivism"[8] have no place in professional or public discourse about obesity.

Dimension	Explicit Bias Trend 2007-2020	Implicit Bias Trend 2007-2020
Sexuality	↓	↓
Race	↓	↓
Skin Tone	↓	↓
Age	↓	↔
Disability	↓	↔
Weight	↓	↑ ↔

Source: Charlesworth & Banaji, 2022, *Psychological Science*

Fig. 1. Trends in explicit and implicit bias 2007 to 2020. (*Data from* Charlesworth TE, Banaji MR. Patterns of implicit and explicit attitudes: IV. change and stability from 2007 to 2020. Psychological Science. 2022;33(9):1347–1371. https://doi.org/10.1177/09567976221084257)

THE LANGUAGE OF PANIC

Substantial literature suggests that much of the public discourse about obesity has served to promote a perception of a moral panic.[9] Academic publications about obesity frequently introduce obesity as a *global crisis*, an *epidemic*, a *pandemic*, or a *syndemic* that is contributing not only to poor health but also to great environmental and economic harm.

Language that aims to heighten the perception of a threat to public and personal health from obesity also often serves to promote a sense of doom and futility. With limited access to effective therapies for this condition, patients often interpret messages about obesity presenting a dire health threat as evidence that they have done grave harm to themselves, increasing their feelings of internalized bias or self-stigma. Internalized stigma is common among people with obesity and is associated with significantly worse health outcomes.[10]

In *What We Don't Talk About When We Talk About Fat*, author Aubrey Gordon describes how this language bombards a person living with obesity:

> *I'm just concerned for your health. I'm concerned for your health, so I have to tell you, again and again, that you're going to die. I'm concerned for your health, so I have to tell you that no one will love you at your size. I'm concerned for your health, so I cannot treat you with basic respect.*[11]

Gordon describes not any single interaction but the cumulative effect of messaging calibrated to heighten the sense of panic about the health effects of obesity. One of the consequences of such catastrophizing language is to energize a fat acceptance movement that has come to view all messaging about obesity with suspicion and to reject the very idea of obesity as a legitimate medical diagnosis.[12]

The stigma of cancer offers a useful illustration of the human reaction to a disease that people view as both harmful and hopeless. For centuries, the stigma of a cancer diagnosis led physicians to avoid any mention of it (or to whisper the term) because of the perception that equated cancer with death.[13] That stigma, although less today than in earlier years, still interferes with preventive care and early diagnosis and can interfere with communication among health-care providers, patients, and families.

Although a diagnosis of obesity is surely different from that of cancer, patients nonetheless view obesity so negatively that they often reject any mention of it, and clinicians are similarly reluctant to discuss obesity with patients.[14]

Thus, the language of panic serves to amplify stigma and to interfere with clinical care for this condition. This is especially regrettable in an era when treatment options are quickly improving.

PEOPLE FIRST

Kyle and Puhl observed that people-first language is not used as frequently in publications about obesity as it is for other diseases that are more generally accepted as a medical diagnosis:

> *Obese is an identity. Obesity is a disease. By addressing the disease separately from the person – and doing it consistently – we can pursue this disease while fully respecting the people affected.*[15]

Kyle and colleagues studied preferences for the use of people-first language in both diabetes and obesity, as well as its relationship to bias and social distance. In an acute exposure, they did not find an effect for the use of person-first language in obesity but they did find that individuals who use people-first language for obesity exhibit less explicit bias toward people with obesity than those who use condition-first language.[16,17]

As a result, the professional and patient organizations that focus on obesity research, advocacy, and clinical care have adopted the use of people-first language in publications related to obesity. In addition, the American Medical Association[18] and the American Academy of Pediatrics[19] have adopted policy statements endorsing this standard.

Recent analyses have shown that adoption of this language in scientific literature has begun but it remains low and inconsistent.[20,21]

WEIGHT LOSS AND OBESITY CARE

The advent of a newer and more effective generation of antiobesity medications (AOMs) has generated an impressive wave of public attention to the subject of obesity and its treatment. However, with this attention has come some considerable attention to the confusion between a medical understanding of obesity, for which these medicines are intended, and cultural notions about body weight, body image, and weight loss.[22,23]

In popular culture, a common presumption is that weight loss is a simple cure for obesity and overweight. And thus, both the public and even health professionals express surprise and skepticism about the fact that AOMs only work to control obesity while patients are taking them. This results from the popular misconception of obesity as a behavioral problem stemming from poor habits that cause weight gain, rather than a complex chronic disease that results from the interaction of environmental triggers in physiologically susceptible individuals.[24]

Even though most health professionals can recognize that obesity is a complex chronic disease, they often describe it as a simple problem of excess weight to be solved by weight loss. However, evidence-based guidelines for obesity treatment are moving away from a simplistic reliance on body mass index (BMI) and weight loss as singular measures for health status. For example, one of the key points of the Canadian Clinical Practice Guideline for Obesity in Adults states this quite clearly:

> *This guideline update reflects substantial advances in the epidemiology, determinants, pathophysiology, assessment, prevention and treatment of obesity, and*

shifts the focus of obesity management toward improving patient-centered health outcomes, rather than weight loss alone.[25]

Confusion of weight loss with obesity treatment makes the adoption of effective strategies for coping with obesity more difficult. It also promotes confusion about the value of new AOMs. Although weight loss might be a short-term goal in obesity treatment, by itself, it is seldom adequate for delivering long-term improvements in health. People who view AOMs as useful simply for short-term weight loss are more likely to find them disappointing because after acute therapy, weight regain is expected. Payers have used the expectation that a short course of therapy should have a permanent effect as a rationale for denying coverage.[26]

As measured by Google Trends[27] data, public interest in "weight loss" is infinitely more prevalent than interest in obesity treatment and 10 times more prevalent than any interest in any reference to "obesity." Even in academic literature, Google Scholar[28] reveals 5 times more references to "weight loss" than to "obesity treatment." Searches for news coverage of new obesity drugs reveal similar disparities in reports that identify them as "weight loss drugs" rather than "obesity drugs."

Persistent use of the terms *weight* and *weight loss* to describe obesity and its treatment frames obesity as a disease of size and appearance rather than one of impaired health. Thus, the confusion about the role and value for obesity treatment persists.

SUMMARY

Language is essential for framing the public and professional understanding of obesity. Historically, the understanding of this complex chronic disease has been inaccurate, dominated by the characterization of it as a simple problem of excess weight caused by poor personal choice and unhealthy behaviors. However, there is a good reason to hope that this is changing. In 2023, the American Heart Association changed its long-standing characterization of high BMI as a health behavior to categorize it instead as biological risk factor for heart disease, analogous to high blood pressure.[29]

To promote better understanding of obesity as an important diagnosis that requires effective clinical care, appropriate language is essential. This includes the elimination of stigmatizing language from both professional and public discourse about obesity. Labeling people who have this disease as "obese" is no more appropriate than it would be to label people with cancer as "cancerous." Furthermore, language that promotes the perception of obesity as a cause for moral panic does not foster an effective response to obesity. Rather, it promotes stigma and interferes with constructive action.

Finally, it is essential to separate the cultural and aesthetic interest in weight loss from the medical management of obesity. An important step toward that end will be to eliminate language that equates weight loss with obesity treatment.

CLINICAL CARE POINTS

- Implicit bias about obesity and people who live with it is an impediment to individual and public health.
- Language serves an important role in shaping the public understanding of obesity.
- Inappropriate language that promotes misinformation, stigma, and ineffective approaches to obesity can thus be a significant health issue.

- Shaping a more effective response to obesity can start with the careful use of language that frames obesity in ways that are scientifically accurate, easily understood, and free from bias.

DISCLOSURE

T.K. Kyle: Personal fees from Boehringer Ingelheim, Novo Nordisk, Nutrisystem, Roman Health Ventures S.Kahan: Consulting fees from Lilly, Novo Nordisk, Vivus. J.Nadglowski: Employment by the Obesity Action Coalition.

REFERENCES

1. Pollack A. A.M.A. recognizes obesity as a disease. The New York Times. June 18, 2013. https://www.nytimes.com/2013/06/19/business/ama-recognizes-obesity-as-a-disease.html. Accessed August 5, 2023.
2. Charlesworth TE, Banaji MR. Patterns of implicit and explicit attitudes: IV. change and stability from 2007 to 2020. Psychol Sci 2022;33(9):1347–71.
3. Puhl RM. Weight stigma and barriers to effective obesity care. Gastroenterol Clin N Am 2023;52(2):417–28.
4. Kersbergen I, Robinson E. Blatant dehumanization of people with obesity. Obesity 2019;27(6):1005–12.
5. Wolsiefer KJ, Mehl M, Moskowitz GB, et al. Investigating the relationship between resident physician implicit bias and language use during a clinical encounter with Hispanic patients. Health Commun 2021;38(1):124–32.
6. Zomorodi M, Monteleone K, Meshkinpour S. Does language shape how we think? NPR 2023;24. https://www.npr.org/2023/02/24/1159075553/does-language-shape-how-we-think. Accessed August 5, 2023.
7. Sharma AM, Kushner RF. A proposed clinical staging system for Obesity. Int J Obes 2009;33(3):289–95.
8. Kyle TK, Nadglowski JF, Nece PM. Recidivism: An artifact of implicit weight bias in obesity research. Obesity 2021;29(8):1237.
9. Mannion R, Small N. On folk devils, moral panics and New Wave Public Health. Int J Health Pol Manag 2019;8(12):678–83.
10. Puhl RM, Lessard LM, Himmelstein MS, et al. The roles of experienced and internalized weight stigma in healthcare experiences: Perspectives of adults engaged in weight management across six countries. PLoS One 2021;16(6). https://doi.org/10.1371/journal.pone.0251566.
11. Gordon A. *What We Don't Talk about When We Talk about Fat.* NY: Penguin Random House; 2022.
12. Parker I. Ob*Sity is a social construct not a disease. Decolonizing Fitness 2021. Available at: https://decolonizingfitness.com/blogs/decolonizing-fitness/ob-sity-is-a-social-construct-not-a-disease. Accessed August 6, 2023.
13. Holland JC, Gooen-Piels J. Historical Perspective. In: Kufe DW, Pollock RE, Weichselbaum RR, et al, editors. Holland-frei cancer medicine. 6th edition. Hamilton (ON): BC Decker; 2003. Available at: https://www.ncbi.nlm.nih.gov/books/NBK12903/.
14. Puhl RM. What words should we use to talk about weight? A systematic review of quantitative and qualitative studies examining preferences for weight-related terminology. Obes Rev 2020;21(6). https://doi.org/10.1111/obr.13008.
15. Kyle TK, Puhl RM. Putting people first in obesity. Obesity 2014;22(5):1211.

16. Kyle TK, Puhl RM, Williams RM, et al. People-First Language, Demographics, and Bias Against Persons with Diabetes or Obesity. Obesity 2013. November 11-16, 2013; Atlanta, Ga. Available at: https://conscienhealth.org/wp-content/uploads/2013/11/People-First-Language-Demographics-and-Bias-Against-Persons-with-Diabetes-or-Obesity-Handout.Final_.pdf.
17. Kyle TK, Puhl RM, Williams RM, et al. People-First Language Is an Indication of Less Explicit Weight Bias. Obesity 2013. November 11-16, 2013; Atlanta, Ga. Available at: https://conscienhealth.org/wp-content/uploads/2013/11/People-First-Language-Is-an-Indication-of-Less-Explicit-Weight-Bias.Handout.Final_.pdf.
18. Person-First Language for Obesity H-440.821. AMA Policy finder. June 2017. Available at: https://policysearch.ama-assn.org/policyfinder/detail/obesity?uri=%2FAMADoc%2FHOD.xml-H-440.821.xml. Accessed August 6, 2023.
19. Pont SJ, Puhl R, Cook SR, et al, SECTION ON OBESITY, OBESITY SOCIETY. Stigma experienced by children and adolescents with obesity. Pediatrics 2017;140(6). https://doi.org/10.1542/peds.2017-3034.
20. Dickinson JK, Bialonczyk D, Reece J, et al. Person-first language in diabetes and obesity scientific publications. Diabet Med 2023. https://doi.org/10.1111/dme.15067. Published online.
21. Fisch C, Whelan J, Evans S, et al. Use of person-centred language among scientific research focused on childhood obesity. Pediatric Obesity 2021;17(5). https://doi.org/10.1111/ijpo.12879.
22. Tirrell M. Doctors urged to move beyond BMI alone as a health measure. CNN 2023. Available at: https://www.cnn.com/2023/06/19/health/bmi-doctors-health-measure-wellness/index.html. Accessed August 6, 2023.
23. Etienne V. Ozempic rebound is real: Doctor says weight gain can be “devastating” after stopping. Peoplemag 2023. Available at: https://people.com/health/ozempic-rebound-is-real-doctor-says-weight-gain-can-be-devastating-after-stopping/. Accessed August 6, 2023.
24. Kaplan LM, Golden A, Jinnett K, et al. Perceptions of barriers to effective obesity care: Results from the National Action Study. Obesity 2017;26(1):61–9.
25. Wharton S, Lau DCW, Vallis M, et al. Obesity in adults: A clinical practice guideline. Can Med Assoc J 2020;192(31). https://doi.org/10.1503/cmaj.191707.
26. As weight loss drugs soar in popularity, many who could benefit can’t get them. NBCNews.com. Accessed August 6, 2023. https://www.nbcnews.com/health/health-news/ozempic-wegovy-weight-loss-drugs-demand-soars-rcna68425.
27. Google trends. https://trends.google.com/trends/. Accessed August 6, 2023.
28. Google scholar. https://scholar.google.com/. Accessed August 6, 2023.
29. Kyle TK. American heart decides obesity isn’t a behavior. ConscienHealth 2022. Available at: https://conscienhealth.org/2022/07/american-heart-decides-obesity-isnt-a-behavior/. Accessed August 6, 2023.

UNITED STATES POSTAL SERVICE®

Statement of Ownership, Management, and Circulation (All Periodicals Publications Except Requester Publications)

1. Publication Title	2. Publication Number	3. Filing Date
GASTROENTEROLOGY CLINICS OF NORTH AMERICA	000 – 279	9/18/23
4. Issue Frequency	**5. Number of Issues Published Annually**	**6. Annual Subscription Price**
MAR, JUN, SEP, DEC	4	$379.00

7. Complete Mailing Address of Known Office of Publication (*Not printer*) (*Street, city, county, state, and ZIP+4®*)
ELSEVIER INC.
230 Park Avenue, Suite 800
New York, NY 10169

Contact Person
Malathi Samayan
Telephone (*Include area code*)
91-44-4299-4507

8. Complete Mailing Address of Headquarters or General Business Office of Publisher (*Not printer*)
ELSEVIER INC.
230 Park Avenue, Suite 800
New York, NY 10169

9. Full Names and Complete Mailing Addresses of Publisher, Editor, and Managing Editor (*Do not leave blank*)

Publisher (*Name and complete mailing address*)
DOLORES MELONI, ELSEVIER INC.
1600 JOHN F KENNEDY BLVD. SUITE 1600
PHILADELPHIA, PA 19103-2899

Editor (*Name and complete mailing address*)
KERRY HOLLAND, ELSEVIER INC.
1600 JOHN F KENNEDY BLVD. SUITE 1600
PHILADELPHIA, PA 19103-2899

Managing Editor (*Name and complete mailing address*)
PATRICK MANLEY, ELSEVIER INC.
1600 JOHN F KENNEDY BLVD. SUITE 1600
PHILADELPHIA, PA 19103-2899

10. Owner (*Do not leave blank. If the publication is owned by a corporation, give the name and address of the corporation immediately followed by the names and addresses of all stockholders owning or holding 1 percent or more of the total amount of stock. If not owned by a corporation, give the names and addresses of the individual owners. If owned by a partnership or other unincorporated firm, give its name and address as well as those of each individual owner. If the publication is published by a nonprofit organization, give its name and address.*)

Full Name	Complete Mailing Address
WHOLLY OWNED SUBSIDIARY OF REED/ELSEVIER, US HOLDINGS	1600 JOHN F KENNEDY BLVD. SUITE 1600 PHILADELPHIA, PA 19103-2899

11. Known Bondholders, Mortgagees, and Other Security Holders Owning or Holding 1 Percent or More of Total Amount of Bonds, Mortgages, or Other Securities. If none, check box → ☐ None

Full Name	Complete Mailing Address
N/A	

12. Tax Status (*For completion by nonprofit organizations authorized to mail at nonprofit rates*) (*Check one*)
The purpose, function, and nonprofit status of this organization and the exempt status for federal income tax purposes:
☒ Has Not Changed During Preceding 12 Months
☐ Has Changed During Preceding 12 Months (*Publisher must submit explanation of change with this statement*)

13. Publication Title: GASTROENTEROLOGY CLINICS OF NORTH AMERICA

14. Issue Date for Circulation Data Below: APRIL 2023

15. Extent and Nature of Circulation			Average No. Copies Each Issue During Preceding 12 Months	No. Copies of Single Issue Published Nearest to Filing Date
a. Total Number of Copies (*Net press run*)			140	132
b. Paid Circulation (*By Mail and Outside the Mail*)	(1)	Mailed Outside-County Paid Subscriptions Stated on PS Form 3541 (*Include paid distribution above nominal rate, advertiser's proof copies, and exchange copies*)	68	70
	(2)	Mailed In-County Paid Subscriptions Stated on PS Form 3541 (*Include paid distribution above nominal rate, advertiser's proof copies, and exchange copies*)	0	0
	(3)	Paid Distribution Outside the Mails Including Sales Through Dealers and Carriers, Street Vendors, Counter Sales, and Other Paid Distribution Outside USPS®	51	46
	(4)	Paid Distribution by Other Classes of Mail Through the USPS (e.g., First-Class Mail®)	8	4
c. Total Paid Distribution [*Sum of 15b (1), (2), (3), and (4)*] ▶			127	120
d. Free or Nominal Rate Distribution (*By Mail and Outside the Mail*)	(1)	Free or Nominal Rate Outside-County Copies included on PS Form 3541	12	11
	(2)	Free or Nominal Rate In-County Copies Included on PS Form 3541	0	0
	(3)	Free or Nominal Rate Copies Mailed at Other Classes Through the USPS (e.g., First-Class Mail)	0	0
	(4)	Free or Nominal Rate Distribution Outside the Mail (*Carriers or other means*)	1	1
e. Total Free or Nominal Rate Distribution (*Sum of 15d (1), (2), (3) and (4)*)			13	12
f. Total Distribution (*Sum of 15c and 15e*) ▶			140	132
g. Copies not Distributed (*See Instructions to Publishers #4 (page #3)*) ▶			0	0
h. Total (*Sum of 15f and g*)			140	132
i. Percent Paid (*15c divided by 15f times 100*) ▶			91.06%	90.91%

* If you are claiming electronic copies, go to line 16 on page 3. If you are not claiming electronic copies, skip to line 17 on page 3.

16. Electronic Copy Circulation	Average No. Copies Each Issue During Preceding 12 Months	No. Copies of Single Issue Published Nearest to Filing Date
a. Paid Electronic Copies ▶		
b. Total Paid Print Copies (Line 15c) + Paid Electronic Copies (Line 16a) ▶		
c. Total Print Distribution (Line 15f) + Paid Electronic Copies (Line 16a) ▶		
d. Percent Paid (Both Print & Electronic Copies) (16b divided by 16c × 100) ▶		

☒ **I certify that 50% of all my distributed copies (electronic and print) are paid above a nominal price.**

17. Publication of Statement of Ownership
☒ If the publication is a general publication, publication of this statement is required. Will be printed in the DECEMBER 2023 issue of this publication.
☐ Publication not required

18. Signature and Title of Editor, Publisher, Business Manager, or Owner
Malathi Samayan - Distribution Controller
Malathi Samayan
Date: 9/18/23

I certify that all information furnished on this form is true and complete. I understand that anyone who furnishes false or misleading information on this form or who omits material or information requested on the form may be subject to criminal sanctions (including fines and imprisonment) and/or civil sanctions (including civil penalties).

9780323940139